Decision Making in Medicine

Decision Making in Medicine:

the practice of its ethics

Edited by Gordon Scorer MBE, MA, MD, FRCS
Surgeon, Hillingdon Hospital and Southall-Norwood Hospitals

and Antony Wing MA, DM, FRCP
Consultant General Physician, St. Thomas' Hospital, London

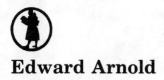

Edward Arnold

© Edward Arnold (Publishers) Ltd. 1979

First published 1979 by
Edward Arnold (Publishers) Ltd
41 Bedford Square, London WC1B 3DQ

British Library Cataloguing in Publication Data
Decision making in medicine.
  1. Medical ethics   2. Medicine – Decision making
  I. Scorer, Charles Gordon   II. Wing, Antony
  174'.2   R724

  ISBN 0–7131–4342–8

Phototypeset in V.I.P. Century Schoolbook by
Western Printing Services Ltd, Bristol
Printed in Great Britain by Pitman Press

Contributors

Caroline Berry PhD(Lond) MB, BS(Lond)
 Senior Registrar, Paediatric Research Unit, Guy's Hospital.
Robert James Berry MA(Cantab), PhD(Lond), DSc(Lond)
 Professor of Genetics in University of London. Head of Genetics
 Department, Royal Free Hospital School of Medicine.
Hugh Handley Bird, MA, MB, BCh(Cantab), MRCGP, DRCOG,
 DCH(Eng)
 General Practitioner, Linton, Kent.
Ralph Colin Evans, BSc, MB, BCh(Wales), FRCP(Ed), DCH(Eng)
 Paediatrician, University Hospital of Wales, Cardiff.
Reginald Frank Robert Gardner, LRCP, LRCS(Ed), FRCOG(Glas)
 Obstetrician and Gynaecologist, Sunderland Hospital Group.
Janet Goodall, MB, ChB(Sheff), FRCP(Ed), DRCOG, DCH(Eng)
 Paediatrician, City General Hospital, Stoke-on-Trent, Staffs.
John Stuart Horner, MB, ChB(Birm), FFCM, DPH(Lond), DIH(Eng)
 Area Medical Officer, Croydon Area Health Authority, Surrey.
Douglas MacGilchrist Jackson, MA, MD(Cantab), FRCS(Eng)
 Senior Clinical Lecturer, University of Birmingham. Surgeon,
 Birmingham Accident Hospital.
Jennifer Tanner Robinson, MB, BS(Lond)
 Housewife and mother.
Charles Gordon Scorer, MBE, MA, MD(Cantab), FRCS(Ed and Eng)
 Surgeon, Hillingdon Hospital, Middlesex.
William Yuille Sinclair, MB, BS(Durh), MRCOG
 Obstetrician and Gynaecologist, Sunderland Hospital Group.
David Anthony Toms, MB, BS(Lond), MRCP(Lond), MRCP Psych,
 DRCOG, DCH(Eng), DPM
 Clinical Teacher, Nottingham University Medical School. Con-
 sultant Psychiatrist, Mapperly Hospital, Nottingham.
Robert Geoffrey Twycross, MA, DM(Oxon), MRCP(Lond)
 Consultant Physician, The Churchill Hospital, Oxford.
David Arthur John Tyrrell, MD(Sheff), FRCP(Lond), FRC Path, FRS
 Deputy Director of Clinical Research Centre and Head of Divi-
 sion of Communicable Diseases, Clinical Research Centre, Har-
 row, Middlesex, and Common Cold Research Unit, Salisbury,
 Wilts.
John Allister Vale, MB, BS(Lond), MRCP(UK)
 Senior Medical Registrar, Guy's Hospital, London.
David John Warren, DPhil(Oxon), BSc(Sheff), BM, BCh(Oxon),
 MRCP(UK)
 Physician, Portsmouth Hospital Group.

Michael Murray Webb-Peploe, MA, MB, BChir(Cantab), FRCP(Lond)
Physician in Charge, Department of Cardiology, St. Thomas'
Hospital, London.
Antony John Wing, MA, DM(Oxon), FRCP(Lond)
Physician, St. Thomas' Hospital, London.

Preface

Within the last three or four decades – that is during the professional life-time of a doctor now nearing his retirement – medical practice has changed radically. Techniques for the doctor's effective intervention have proliferated. The better informed public for whom he works has become more critical. There has been a revolution in his conditions of service. But, at heart, medical practice remains – and will continue to remain – the same. The personal consultation between doctor and patient will always be central as long as illness is the lot of mankind. From the doctor's point of view the most significant change is that he now has to take many more difficult decisions with far-reaching consequences. This has made medical ethics a subject of very great importance.

Not long ago it was necessary to ransack the shelves of the older medical libraries to find a book of any kind on *Medical Ethics*. By chance, a copy of one written in 1803 by Thomas Percival under that title might be there. But on perusal it would be found to contain advice to doctors on how to live amicably and courteously with their colleagues by adhering to some simple principles of conduct. In addition it gave common-sense guidance in methods of practice suggesting how clinical work might be better organized to make it more efficient. Much of what was then called ethics we might today consider to be etiquette. It was – and still is – highly relevant, but our concern in this book is with broader issues.

Ethics, in its fuller sense, is now being widely discussed both within and outside medical circles. This is primarily because of the extent to which the doctor is being asked to intervene in, or to modify, the human body. The kind of active intervention, which has been made possible by modern medical techniques, raises many new ethical questions. It is the doctor who must decide whether or not to carry out investigations or institute treatment or perform operations on his patient. He must weigh the inconvenience and risk against the gain for the individual. He should also take account of the effects (both immediate and long-term) of his decision on society as a whole.

The science of genetics, for example, offers the possibility of reducing the numbers of, or even eliminating, certain congenital disorders but is the price to be paid in the threat to the liberty of the parents too high? Is scientific feasibility the only limit to interference with life processes? Modern surgery has become so exact and modern anaesthesia so safe and acceptable that operations have largely lost the terrors they used to hold. By what criteria shall we judge when to offer and when to withhold surgical skills which are being sought merely for personal or social reasons? Again, pharmacological advances in the relief of mental and physical distress and in the control of moods are now very rapid. Personal expectation of help in all sorts of emotional situations has become common. But the distinction between what is truly medical need and what represents a surrender of proper personal responsibility has become blurred. To prescribe, or not to prescribe, is often an ethical problem not a clinical one.

Not unconnected with technical advances is the increasing control which the State now holds over the Medical Profession. None will deny that good medical services ought to be available to all citizens. However, medical resources are becoming very expensive. The State, which holds the purse strings, is responsible for taking practical decisions about national priorities. The reality of financial restraint means that it is not possible to apply all the advances of scientific medicine. It is also resulting in an ever widening gap between medical care in the affluent countries and in developing nations. On what grounds shall we decide who shall receive scarce resources available? This is an ethical and practical problem, but one which the medical profession cannot escape and over the last decade we have come to realize it is a key issue in the medical services of the future.

We live in a shrinking world. The individual must be restrained from damaging the interests of his fellow-men by his own greed and acquisitiveness. The collective 'good' is widely accepted to be more important than that of the individual. But who now protects the individual when the powers of the group become oppressive? The doctor has hitherto been trusted as the patient's confidant, counsellor and friend, and yet he may find that at the bidding of some pressure group, or of the State itself, he is expected to do what in conscience he opposes. Legislation, or political or financial constraint, may mean that he can be called upon to advise or to act in a way which is contrary to what he believes to be in the best interests of his patient. Who then shall decide what is ethically right?

The editors have chosen from a wide range of medical problems those which at the present time, and for the forseeable future, seem most likely to offer subjects for ethical debate. Contributors are experts in their own fields. They all write from a busy professional involvement and are therefore able both to see the changing circumstances of practice and to know where they and their patients are experiencing the pressures of difficult decisions.

The answer to such difficult questions cannot be found simply by looking at the problems and listening to what the patient and our colleagues and our friends have to say. We have to bring something to the problems from outside. We need to apply our understanding of man and of his place in society, of personal responsibility and the meaning of health. There is no way forward by repeatedly adjusting ethical decision to changing public opinion while in the meantime we try to keep pace with the ever new technical possibilities available to us.

The viewpoint of the writers is in agreement with the outlook and philosophy of the Profession as it developed over the latter part of the nineteenth and early part of the twentieth centuries. Most doctors in this period were deeply influenced by the Greek Medicine of Hippocrates and Galen and by the Judaeo-Christian traditions of Western Europe. From this strong stock there has grown so much that is best in current medical practice. However, since the first world war, there has been a progressive decline in the influence of religion in society and an increased secularization of education and public life. After the second world war the technological revolution in communication and the control of life greatly accelerated changes in public opinion and accepted standards of conduct.

The thinking of the profession has tended to follow the processes of disintegration. Fewer of those becoming doctors today have been educated in the knowledge of the former truths which gave wisdom and strength to the medical profession and bred confidence in their patients. In putting this book together we have, therefore, particularly had in mind junior medical students and younger doctors, for it is they who often meet the ethical problems in urgent reality and may be ill-prepared to face them.

It is the opinion of the editors and contributors that the principles and insights bequeathed to us from the past need to be retained and reaffirmed. They are too valuable to lose for they have a continuing relevance and offer the best promise for the further development of modern Medicine.

Hillingdon Hospital   C.G.S.
St. Thomas' Hospital   A.J.W.

Contents

1

The Moral Values, Law and Religion
Gordon Scorer

In any stable, progressive society there must always be a general agreement on what is right and what is wrong in human behaviour. Without such agreement dissension and disorder occur to an extent which soon becomes intolerable.

The most elementary aspects of order relate to the preservation and protection of life, respect for marriage and the family and the safeguarding of property. If a promise is made it must be kept; if a service is rendered, it should be acknowledged; furthermore, if damage is done, reparation needs to be made. No community can thrive without a general acceptance that living together involves keeping certain unwritten rules.

On such a foundation other general concepts of what is right and what is wrong will be built. These will include provisions for the development of trade, for the protection of privacy, for facilitating communication, for the maintenance of order and for the restraint of evil-doers. In this way law is written down and codified to preserve those institutions which man finds necessary for peace and for progress and a system of acceptable human conduct is established which is passed on to the next generation.

The part played by law and its sanctions may change from time to time. Some may wish to try to enforce conformity to particular standards, others prefer to keep a less rigid control in order to allow for desirable changes to occur. If a particular law loses the support of a majority in the community it will need to be appropriately changed, but what must not be allowed to happen – because of its damaging effect – is for a nation to lose confidence in its own behaviour patterns and allow men and women to do what they please. That will lead sooner or later to a disruption of social life and, possibly, to violence requiring government by regulation and decree to replace government by general consent. Law and order will then need to be imposed by force in order to protect life and property and maintain communication.

Morals and Ethics

The concept that some actions are good and others evil is to be found among all peoples everywhere. When man has to choose between right and wrong he makes a *moral* decision. General agreement in a community on what is right and wrong in human conduct constitutes an ethical system.

1

The word 'moral' (from the Latin *mos, moris* meaning manners) describes a particular type of human behaviour. The word 'mores' (not appearing in the older dictionaries) is applied to the characteristic manners of a society and the customs which support them.

Although moral is basically a neutral word it has extended its meaning so that moral conduct is regarded as right conduct and immoral as wrong. Human nature being what it is, the word has developed a slightly derogatory meaning. A 'moralizer' is one who is dogmatic in opinion or censorious in judgment of another's activities, and, in contrast, an immoral person may be described as one who has offended against the commonly held code of sexual behaviour. Perhaps it is in this denigrating sense that some doctors will advocate that morals and Medicine should never be mixed, although that is an impossibility. For instance, a doctor not infrequently has to consider what to do when faced with a clinical problem which affects human life or liberty or privacy. In such a case his decision will probably be moral as well as medical.

On the other hand, the word 'ethics' (from the Greek *ethos* meaning customs, habits) has obtained a more theoretical sense in modern usage. It relates to the precepts which should control moral behaviour. It is the science which is concerned with the nature and grounds of moral obligations, distinguishing what is right from wrong and the reasons for it.

It is obvious that between different societies, whose history, culture and language are distinctive, there will be different points of view on what constitutes right and wrong in human behaviour.

The science of ethics, therefore, aims to define the grounds and validity of the various systems of principles and secondary rules governing conduct and duty. There are a number of ethical systems in the world today, chiefly deriving from the religious beliefs of ethnic groups; each system presupposes a particular view of the world, of human life, human destiny and human relationships.

Religion as the Source of Ethics

How then are ethical systems derived? They arise out of man's understanding of the world in which he lives and the role he ought to be playing in it. He sees his relationship to his environment and to his fellow men and women, to the past and to the future in a particular way. He decides in agreement with others and usually because of the influence of wise, far-sighted and strong leaders that there are things which he ought to do and others which he ought not to do, actions which are right and those which are wrong.

It is the great religions of the world, with their honoured leaders, which have, for the most part, shaped the ethical thinking of the nations, but a visit to a Hindu, a Muslim or a Buddhist land will soon show the difference in personal and communal behavior when com-

pared with a Western European nation with its Christian background. To live in a family, to witness a marriage or be present at a
death, to work in a business or trade in one of these other cultures
reveals a system of ethics different from our own. There are obviously
broad areas of agreement common to any society but there are differences of attitude and understanding surrounded and supported by
customs which are centuries old and deeply rooted.

The very fact that there are now established and growing in our
own country many communities adhering to one or other of these
great religions presents the possibility of ethical conflict. We now
live, as it is said, in a pluralist society. In medical practice, as we give
service to those of creeds or colour different from our own, problems
will often arise because of differences of moral behaviour and custom.

In the Western world our own ethical system has been largely built
up on a Judaeo-Christian foundation. The influence of Greek and
Roman thought has also been considerable and, over the years, there
have been other minor influences. In the past two centuries, however,
new and powerful ideas have joined the main stream, challenging
and tending to disintegrate the Judaeo-Christian concepts. The
moral outlook of Western nations, their institutions and their laws
are now undergoing major changes. We live today not only in a
pluralist society but in one of ethical uncertainty and confusion. But
let us first examine the foundations.

Judaean and Christian Ethics

Israel's ethical system comes from the Law given on Sinai by God
the Creator. It occupies a unique place in the thought of the Old
Testament and the beginning of the New Testament. The teaching of
Christ arises out of the matrix of the Jewish rabbinical training and
cannot be fully understood except in the context of 'the Law of God'
and the worship of the synagogue. 'What great nation', said Moses
Israel's appointed leader, 'is there that has a god so near it as the Lord
our God is to us, whenever we call upon Him? And what great nation
is there, that has statutes and ordinances so righteous as all this Law
which I set before you this day?' (Deuteronomy 4, 7 & 8).

The heart of the Law, as we know it today, is to be found in the Ten
Commandments, the Decalogue. This is in part religious – a primary
duty owed to God – in part moral precept and in part legal duty. In
those days these three ideas, religion, morals and law – which we now
tend often to treat separately – were intermingled and this can be
seen constantly in the Old Testament writings. Religious and moral
instruction was to be carefully passed on from one generation to the
next – 'these words which I command you shall be on your heart and
you shall teach them diligently to your children, and shall talk of
them when you sit in your house and when you walk in the way, and
when you lie down, and when you rise'. (Deuteronomy 6, 6 & 7).

All through its history Israel tended to forget the Law, to depart from its God and to follow the more attractive and less rigorous worship of the pagan nations around them. At times – as in the reign of Josiah – the Scrolls of the Law were rediscovered, it was again accepted and obeyed and the people returned to a true worship. Moral uprightness came into its own. With the great prophets of the eighth and seventh centuries BC, Hosea, Amos, Isaiah and Jeremiah, the Jews came to view God as the God of the whole earth, ruling according to the universal principle of righteousness and goodness.

The Law remained at the heart of Judaism and remains there today. When Jesus Christ began His teaching He made plain that as a Jew and as Israel's Messiah He was absolutely loyal to the Law. 'Think not', He said, 'that I have come to abolish the Law and the Prophets; I have not come to abolish them but to fulfil them'. (Mat. 5, 17).

But the Christian ethic differs in its emphasis from that of Judaism. Rather than observation of the detailed prescriptions of the Divine Law, it calls for a spirit of obedience to the principles enshrined within it. Christ's teaching is squarely based on the Law and the Prophets but He shifts the emphasis from conformity to the letter of the many detailed rules to a new inner attitude expressive of the spirit behind them. He alters the motivation for keeping the Law from a negative attitude of fear for the Law-giver to a response of gratitude to Him for His loving kindness. Mere outward conformity will not suffice; it is the response of the heart that matters. This is readily seen in His Summary of the Law of which all the elements are taken from Israel's *Torah*. To take the Ten Commandments as an example, Christ summarizes Table ī (Commandments 1–4) as, 'You shall love the Lord your God with all your heart and with all your soul and with all your mind and with all your strength' (Mark *12*, 30). Similarly, Table īī (Commandments 5–10) is summarized as 'You shall love your neighbour as yourself' (Mark *12*, 31) or, on another occasion, 'Whatever you wish that men would do to you, do so to them; for this is the Law and the Prophets' (Matthew 7, 12). Hence, Christ's teaching on right living becomes possible because the motive in all relationships both with the Law-giver and with fellow citizens, is to be based on gratitude and love.

Greek and Roman Ideals

If Jewish ethics are primarily religious and concerned with man's duty to fulfil the divine law of righteousness, Greek ethics were philosophical and concerned with human achievement. Socrates, Plato and Aristotle sought to understand and to analyse what were regarded as moral virtues and how human perfection could thereby be attained. Such thinking developed in two directions. The Epicureans emphasized the pleasure of intellect and friendship, whereas the Stoics dwelt on the importance of right judgments and decisions based on reason.

The Greek ideal became embodied in perfection of personality. 'Man is the measure of all things' is an aphorism attributed to Protagoras of Abdera (480 BC). It was the pursuit of what was good and true that mattered and this beauty of character extended also to the body. Health was the highest possession, for only the healthy man was a complete human being; disease made him inferior. But the Greek contribution to civilization – and to posterity – covered a wide field in poetry and drama, in architecture and sculpture as well as mathematics, science and medicine.

The Romans, much influenced by Greek thought, were a practical people. They were concerned for material prosperity and happiness and developed a legal system to regulate the conditions of life to this end.

Renaissance and Reformation

The importance of Greek thought lies in its enormous influence on the Medieval Church and subsequently at the Renaissance. Aristotle is said to have had 'an incalculable influence on Christian theology and ethics'.[1] Thus Thomas Aquinas (1224–1274) made use of Aristotle's writings in building up his own ethical system and in particular his concept of 'natural law' (which considers that man, unaided by religious beliefs, can attain to a partial understanding of God's eternal laws). The natural virtues in man had to be supplemented by the theological virtues of faith, hope and love. More detailed rules and examples were added in later centuries. Thomism remains at the centre of the ethical teaching of the Roman Catholic church today.

The Renaissance was a change in direction of thought and action in Western Europe. It lifted the nations out of their medieval mould with its confined and ecclesiastically dominated outlook. The recovery of Greek and Roman ideals contributed substantially to this change. Man, it was realized, was important for his own sake. He could improve his lot by cultured and intelligent living. The physical world around him was worthy of investigation. And this new self assurance was made effective and was disseminated not only as a result of the invention of printing but because of the new possibilities to travel even to the world's ends. Such 'humanism' owed much to the fresh study of the intellectual and artistic achievements of the Greeks and the political and legal prowess of the Romans.

It was far more than a mere revival of classical Greek and Roman culture. It was a determination by thinking men to escape from the narrow confines of authoritarian tradition, to break the limitations imposed by Church and State and to experiment, observe and deduce without prejudice or dogma. This philosophical revolution with its demands for freedom of thought, for a new standard of human dignity, for logical proof instead of credulous acceptance, for experimental observation in place of blind dogma, resulted in revolutions in the fields of theology, astronomy, anatomy and physiology.

But the rebirth was religious as well as secular. Erasmus, the prince of Renaissance scholars, carried his Greek New Testament around Europe. William Tyndale, at the cost of his life, translated and published the Bible into the language of the English people. 'The power of biblical-revelation passed from the priests to the people, from Latin torpor into living common speech'.[2] Men and women began again to realize that laws of righteousness and the truths of the Gospel of Christ were for them personally. The ethical impact of these events was profound and continues to this day. Despite a bitterly divided church and fierce controversy which continued for over a century the nations of the West were agreed in their determination to try to build a Christian civilization, incorporating man's expanding powers.

Reaction and reform have since alternated, manners have fluctuated between the extravagant and the prim, and morals between licentiousness and an over-rigid self-discipline. But always at intervals there has been a return to the basic reforming religious motivation for personal and social ethics. The evangelical revivals of Wesley and Whitfield in the eighteenth century transformed our nation's behaviour patterns. The nineteenth century Evangelicals, relying on the same authority, were foremost in applying their ethical beliefs to the relief of human oppression wherever they saw it.

The New Humanism

The Humanism of the Renaissance was essentially Christian and it had no difficulty in accommodating itself to the new discoveries of man's insignificant place in the physical universe. God's greatness and His revelation of Himself to Man seemed all the more impressive. But, as man became more aware of his own resources and learnt that he could control and manipulate his environment for his own use, he became increasingly self-confident. The new Humanism is self-centred and self-assured. It sees man as a rational being, master of the world, with unlimited capacity for progress and needing to be uncluttered by any authoritarian dogmas or ideas of supernatural revelation. On the other hand it attracts idealistic intellectuals and, on the other, it is favoured by those who are anxious to ameliorate the lot of people through social adjustment. It places its faith in what it believes is the innate goodness and adaptibility of man but it turns a blind eye to his incorrigible selfishness.

In the twentieth century the Existential concept of man, negative in so many of its effects on previously accepted standards, has rapidly gained ground. It is a reaction against reason, claiming that reason is too superficial. It asserts that it is what man is in himself that matters – his deep feelings and his subjective experiences. It is the 'philosophy' of man by himself, rejecting the precepts of the past which tell him what he ought to do and looking to the future with a completely open mind.

Both modern Humanism and Existentialism are to be found in many forms today. They are alike in opposing any religious view, as at least an unnecessary encumbrance but more often as a serious impediment to man's development of his true self. In this world man is the measure of all things. Religion, if it is to be tolerated at all, must be relegated to the area of private opinion and should not obtrude on the practical matters of organized living.

In their world-view man is at the summit of the biological evolutionary scale. He is self-conscious and free to control his own destiny. Biological change is mechanical and extraordinarily slow, but social and ethical changes offer limitless possibilities – hence their enthusiasm for reform (or revolution) in society. Broadly speaking the ethical principles favoured are utilitarian, that is to say, what offers the greatest happiness to the greatest numbers and what leads to a reduction of human physical suffering. Such views, however, are tragically naive, for they do not take adequate account of human nature as it really is with its self-centred and acquisitive propensities. Man may know very well what he ought to do but so often he finds himself incapable of doing it.

The Current Ethical Uncertainty

Many of the ethical principles and rules of conduct which used to govern Western Nations have now been by-passed or allowed to lapse. The Judaeo-Christian heritage which formed the basis of civilization over some 1500 years is being forsaken, but without the foundation the superstructure cannot endure. The various humanist creeds of today give us no secure basis on which to build, so it is no wonder that ethical uncertainty and – in some areas – moral anarchy prevail. Into this setting have come peoples from Eastern nations whose religious thinking and ethnic origin is very different from our own. Their beliefs too need to be taken into account in determining our future way of life – for a nation cannot be divided within itself if its well-being is to be maintained.

Because previous standards have now been largely abandoned, the laws which protected our ancient social institutions have, in recent years, had to be progressively relaxed to accommodate to public opinion and to fall into line with the broadly humanist thinking of our people. Thus, three major concepts, which for centuries past were embodied in the ethical thinking of our leaders and people and fixed in our customs, are now openly questioned. All of them concern the medical practitioner in his daily work. These are, the sanctity of human life, the ideal of permanent monogamy and the necessity to protect and support family life. Other concepts such as the confidentiality of information about persons, the degrees to which the State may dictate to the individual his manner of living, and the rights and wrongs of withdrawing labour are constantly brought into the arena of public debate.

Religion, Law and Morals

We live at a time when the relationship between religion and law is confused and the influence of each on personal conduct is often denied. But law remains a powerful weapon even though at the moment there is much contradictory thinking about it. At one and the same time we oppose its interference in our lives and yet clamour for new laws to control this or that form of conduct of which we disapprove. Judaism, Christianity and Islam are the three great monotheistic religions. Hinduism and Buddhism are both religious faiths which place ulitimate reality outside man himself. But modern Humanism, in all its varieties, rejects any supernatural elements, and as a result allows man to usurp the place of God. When it becomes fully institutionalized and organized it pervades every aspect of man's life, including his thought. It is, in some senses, also a religion, but a false one for the State becomes as a god. But here, by implication, it is only in his relationship to the State that the human individual has value and his life has meaning. The possibilities of exploitation of the individual by the State become limitless.

Religion, law and morality essentially belong together. It is not possible to separate them from one another for long. Many, however, consider that religion concerns our dealings with God and is purely a private and personal matter, whereas law defines and controls our dealings with our fellows. So law in many respects today no longer arises from religious concepts or from 'natural justice'; it is simply an expression of the arbitrary will of the governing power. Laws are therefore made to keep order in society for the benefit of the whole community; the propagation of private morality is anti-social and must be suspended as an unacceptable intrusion. The situation is muddled.

In an Earl Grey Memorial Lecture in 1953, Lord Justice Denning made these comments – 'The severance has, I think, gone too far. Although religion, law and morals can be separated, they are nevertheless still very much dependent on one another. Without religion there can be no morality: and without morality there can be no law'.[3]

Lord Devlin (1965) made the same point about the way in which morals and religion are inextricably joined. 'Outside Christendom', he said, 'other standards derive from other religions. None of these moral codes can claim any validity except by virtue of the religion on which it is based. Old Testament morals differ in some respects from New Testament morals. . . . Between the great religions of the world, of which Christianity is only one, there are much wider differences. It may or may not be right for the State to adopt one of these religions as the truth, to found itself upon its doctrines, and to deny to any of its citizens the liberty to practise any other. If it does, it is logical that it should use the secular law wherever it thinks it necessary to enforce the divine. If it does not, it is illogical that it should concern itself with morals as such. But if it leaves matters of religion to private judgment it should logically leave matters of morals also'.[4]

Which Way?

Western society, in recent decades, has moved towards a materialistic and humanist view of life. This humanism, in its popular materialistic form, is a doctrine which denies the existence of any supernatural or spiritual reality; it teaches that mind is simply an expression of matter and a product of material organization. The morality deriving from such philosophy-become-'religion' places emphasis on the acquisition, retention and development of material resources for man's personal benefit as being the greatest good. The law-maker (the State) then becomes supremely concerned with economic issues, the control of wealth and its distribution and the balancing of the rights of one group against another.

Those matters which most concern man's spirit have, in consequence, been swamped by the rising tide of ambition to improve his material prosperity. Man sees himself free only in so far as he can break loose from the limitations of poverty which prevent his personal enjoyment of 'doing his own thing'. But such individualism leads to a break-down of social cohesion without which no community of people can either flourish or progress. We have to return to the fact that the world in which we live, and our own biological endowment, demand of us a certain ordered pattern of life – an ethical system – without which civilization falls apart. The influence of these recent changes in thought is very evident in medical practice and goes a long way towards explaining the grave problems which the Profession now faces.

The dismantling of the old ideals of society has gone too far. Important elements in the foundations have been weakened. Standards of respect for others and mutual trust and willing service have been drastically eroded. Honesty and integrity have declined. We have come full circle and are again considering moral behaviour. Such morality takes its origin from religion – true religion. And a true religion is one which accords with man's highest ideals for himself and most enhances the welfare both of individuals *and* of the community as a whole. So the support society needs is not that of government statutes – ever-increasing in number – which minutely control our individual and communal economic and commercial activities (necessary though some of them may be) but laws arising from true moral values which safeguard our vital institutions. By this alone can we thrive.

Let the last word be with Lord Denning. 'What does it all come to? Surely this, that if we seek truth and justice we cannot find it by argument and debate, nor by reading and thinking, but only by the maintenance of true religion and virtue. Religion concerns the spirit in man whereby he is able to recognize what is truth and what is justice; whereas law is only application, however imperfectly, of truth and justice in our every day affairs. If religion perishes in the land, truth and justice will also. We have already strayed too far from the faith of our fathers. Let us return to it, for it is the only thing that can save us'.[5]

References

1. Aristotle from Macquarrie, J. (Ed.) (1967) *A Dictionary of Christian Ethics*. London, S.C.M. Press.
2. From *Henry the Eighth*. by F. Hackett.
3. Denning, A. (1953) *The Changing Law*. London, Stevens and Sons.
4. Devlin, P. (1965) *The Enforcement of Morals*. Oxford University Press.
5. Op. cit. p. 122.

Further Reading

Baelz, P. (1977) *Ethics and Belief*. London, Sheldon Press.
Henson, Hensley (1936) *Christian Morality: Natural, Developing, Final*. Oxford, Clarendon Press.
Kitwood, T. (1970) *What is Human*. London, Intervarsity Press.
Macquarrie, J. (Ed.) (1967) *A Dictionary of Christian Ethics*. London, S.C.M. Press.
Mitchell, B. (1970) *Law, Morality and Religion in a Secular Society*. London, Oxford University Press.
Temple, William (1936) *Christianity in Thought and Practice*. London, S.C.M Press.
Thielicke, H. (1968) *Theological Ethics*. London, A. & C. Black.

2

The Medical Profession
Michael Webb-Peploe

All professions, whether Medicine, Law or Accountancy – to name but a few – have certain characteristics in common. Their work involves a person to person contact with interchange of information (often confidential) between the professional man and the one who asks for his help. A fee for service may be freely negotiated between the two.

Anybody aspiring to membership of a profession is required to undertake a formal period of training (which often has an element of apprenticeship) and pass certain qualifying examinations before he is allowed to offer his services to the public.

The members of the profession agree to uphold certain ethical standards. Professional disciplinary bodies exist, charged with the maintenance of these standards and granted limited powers to punish those who flout them. It is of interest that in the United Kingdom these regulatory bodies (whether the General Medical Council, the Bar Council, the Ecclesiastical Courts, or the Press Council) are all independent of the apparatus of the civil law courts.

Such in brief are the characteristics which distinguish a profession from other occupations, but, as we shall see later, some of these time-honoured ideas have recently been questioned.

History of the Medical Profession

'The longer you can look back, the further you can look forward', said Winston Churchill when addressing the Royal College of Physicians in March 1944. In order to understand the present structure and stance of the medical profession, and especially in order to anticipate future trends, some knowledge of the past is essential.

The earliest regulation of medical practice is to be found in the Babylonian laws of Hammurabi (2200 BC).[1] Eight out of the two hundred and eighty-two sections dealt with the fee scales of physicians, graded according to the social status of the patient, for example 'if the doctor shall treat a gentleman and shall open an abscess with a bronze knife and shall preserve the eye of the patient, he shall receive ten shekels of silver. If the patient is a slave, his master shall pay two shekels of silver'. That there might be a debit account for an unfortunate or incompetent doctor is shown by the following rule: 'If the doctor shall open an abscess with a bronze knife and shall kill the patient or shall destroy the sight of the eye, his

11

hands shall be cut off.' This *lex talionis* was practised by Babylonians, Persians and Jews.

The keystone of ancient Egyptian pathology was the idea of devil possession, and medical papyri such as the Eber's Papyrus[2] are plentifully sprinkled with spells and incantations to be used with the remedies. Priest and physician were for centuries one and the same. The failure to distinguish between the physical and the mental or spiritual aspects of disease explains the ancient Egyptians' inability to study the structural changes underlying organic disease, despite the opportunities for *post mortem* examination which was part of the process of embalming.

Greece and Rome

With the Greeks, Medicine separated itself from magic, refusing to be blindly guided by superstition or by rule of thumb. They began to seek out the causes of observed natural phenomena including the phenomena of human physiology and pathology. The great legacy of the Greek philosophers was their insistence on genuine enquiry, their encouragement of critical thought, their demand for proof based on the logical argument and their investigation into causes for the sake of knowledge alone, whether that knowledge could yield immediate practical results or not.

Small wonder then that the ethical code devised by the physicians of Cos and ascribed to Hippocrates[3] (about 400 BC) has been generally accepted without serious questioning until the early part of this century. This code, devised and voluntarily subscribed to by doctors themselves, was probably the work of a sect called the Pythagoreans but how much influence it had on Greek physicians in general cannot be known. It contains the following four major principles:

1) The aim of the doctor should be to advance the profession rather than the individual practitioner: hence no advertising, no enticing away of another doctor's patients, no derogatory remarks about the abilities of colleagues were allowed.

2) Medical knowledge or privilege must never be used to injure but always to help the patient. Life was to be preserved and its destruction by abortion or by drugs was not permitted. Any new discovery must be made available freely to all.

3) Specialist assistance must be called in whenever it was in the best interests of the patient.

4) Professional secrecy must be maintained. A doctor should not disclose without the consent of the patient information which he has obtained in the course of his professional relationship.

Admirable though the Greek spirit of scientific enquiry was, their attitude towards the sick patient left much to be desired. They so exalted the healthy and sound body that disease became a mark of inferiority. Only if a sick man's condition showed likelihood of improvement could he hope for the continued care of the physician or any consideration from society. In exalting the healthy and the sound, the Greek world showed neither compassion nor organized care for the weak and disabled.

Although the Romans were content to leave the practice of medicine and surgery to the Greeks, widespread quackery and medical malpractice forced them to organize medical teaching and medical services for the poor and for their armed forces. Public physicians, or archiatri, were appointed to attend the poor and to supervise medical practice within their area. They were paid a good annual salary 'in order that they may honourably serve the poor rather than basely grovel before the rich'.[4]

Mediaeval Medicine

After the fall of the Roman empire, Medicine followed two distinct and divergent paths which went their separate ways for five hundred years before coming together again in the School of Salerno. On the one hand there were the Arabs who constructed their system of Medicine on the foundation left by the Greeks, but who added their own original observations (notably in the fields of epidemic fevers, eye disease and pharmacology). On the other hand there was the Medicine practised by the mediaeval monasteries. It can be argued that although monastic Medicine made no great scientific contribution to the advancement of the medical profession, it did make a very great contribution to its humanitarian aspect.

With Christianity the significance of disease changed, and so did the position of the sick man in society. The early Christians no longer viewed disease solely as a punishment for sin, but rather as a discipline to be patiently borne and endured. The sick person was no longer abandoned as sinful or inferior, but instead, in response to Christ's command to heal the sick, he was given care and nursing in the monastery hospice, some of which later became famous university hospitals.

At Salerno,[5] after five centuries of comparative stagnation in the widely scattered monasteries of Christendom and in the cities of the vast Moslem Empire, medical learning became established on a sound basis. According to legend, the school was founded by 'four masters': Elinus the Jew, Pontus the Greek, Adale the Arab and Salernus the Latin.[6] This legend underlines two important and novel features of the school: first that it was open to all, irrespective of language and nationality and, second, that it was a lay foundation. No one could proceed to the study of Medicine at Salerno until he had attained the age of twenty-one years, had proved his legitimacy, and had studied logic for three years. The medical course lasted for five years with an additional year of practice under the supervision of an elder practitioner. The candidate, having passed the examinations, took the oath to uphold the school, to attend the poor gratis, to administer no noxious drug, to teach nothing false, and not to keep an apothecary's shop. He then received a ring, a laurel wreath, a book, and the kiss of peace, after which he was entitled to call himself Magister or Doctor and to practise Medicine. This first attempt to co-ordinate the teaching of Medicine without any restriction as to religion or nationality, and to grant degrees only after a definite course of study and the passing of an examination was soon copied by other medical schools set up at Montpellier, Bologna, Paris and Padua. The existence of such medical schools provided the necessary organizational framework for the rapid expansion of knowledge that occurred at the time of the Renaissance.

After the Renaissance

The Renaissance began in Italy about the end of the fourteenth century, and reached its climax some two hundred years later. With the spread of the new learning (aided by the invention of printing) came a new concern with standards of medical practice. Thomas Linacre had noted that too often the practice of Medicine lay in the hands of illiterate monks or of charlatans. In 1518 he obtained from Henry VIII letters patent for a body of regular physicians which later (1551) became the Royal College of Physicians of London. This body was empowered to decide who should practise within the city or within a radius of seven miles round it, and to examine and license practitioners throughout the kingdom. Thomas Vicary in 1540 was instrumental in securing the Royal Assent to a union of the guilds of barber surgeons and surgeons. This Act declared that surgeons should no longer be barbers, and that barbers should restrict their surgery to dentistry. The new Company was empowered to impose fines upon unlicensed practitioners in London, and was entitled to dissect the bodies of two executed criminals each year to further their knowledge of anatomy.

In Scotland in 1505 the surgeons and barbers successfully petitioned the Town Council of Edinburgh for a 'Seal of Cause' conferring upon the Incorporation of Barber Surgeons the sole right of practising within the burgh and of examining candidates who wished to join them to ensure that they could read and write and had adequate knowledge of 'the anatomy, nature, and complexion of man's body'. In 1599 Peter Lowe obtained from King James VI a charter for the faculty of Physicians and Surgeons of Glasgow. In addition to examining candidates and controlling practice in and around Glasgow, the faculty had as one of its original functions the provision of free treatment for the poor ('to give council to puir dissisit folk gratis').

The seventeenth century was a period of intense intellectual activity in the arts and sciences. In his 'Novum Organum' (1620), Francis

Bacon had urged men to abandon the four 'idols' – accepted authority, popular opinion, legal bias, and personal prejudice, and to replace them by the inductive method of reasoning based on experience.[7] The brilliant investigators of that era (Harvey, the Dutch anatomists, the pioneer microscopists, the Oxford physiologists Boyle, Hooke, Lower and Mayow) put this advice into practice. There were those, however, so intoxicated by the new discoveries that they sought to explain all the phenomena of health and disease by regarding the body as a machine (the 'iatro-physical' or 'iatro-mechanical' school), or as a test-tube containing a series of chemical processes (the 'iatro-chemical' school).

It was Thomas Sydenham, the greatest clinician of the seventeenth century, who administered a much needed corrective to the far-fetched theorizing of these two schools, and who restored the sick patient to his rightful place at the centre of medical attention. 'Anatomy, botany, nonsense!', he is reported to have said to Sir Hans Sloane. 'No, young man, go to the bedside; there alone you can learn disease'.[8]

Sydenham's ethical principles which were responsibility and accountability to 'the Supreme Judge', unselfish devotion of skills and talents in the service of suffering humanity, the great value to be placed on human life, true compassion based on the recognition by the physician that he is no better and no different from his patient, can be traced directly to his Christian beliefs. Not for nothing has he been called 'the English Hippocrates', and his views have greatly influenced those who came after him.

Another physician of this era whose writings have continued to impress succeeding generations was Thomas Browne of Norwich. In Osler's words[9] 'Mastery of self, devotion to duty, deep interest in human beings; these best of all lessons may be gleaned from the writings of Sir Thomas Browne'.

The Dawn of Modern Ethics

It was at the end of the eighteenth century that medical ethics began to take a recognizable form. Practice at that time was notable for the wrangling and personal abuse between physicians, often expressed in scurrilous writings. Each man acted more or less as he chose with little regard for his colleagues. Some hospitals were notorious for the internal friction among their medical staff. In 1772 John Gregory, Professor of the Practice of Physic in Edinburgh, published a series of lectures for medical students entitled *Lectures on the Duties and Qualifications of a Physician*.[10] In it he describes the qualities of a good physician, his humanity, humility and truthfulness, his care of the hopeless case, his manners and his dress and other practical matters. Medicine he said is 'a liberal profession whose object is the life and health of the human species, a profession to be exercised by gentlemen of honour and ingenuous manners'.

Change did not come immediately for the old medical individualism remained rampant for some years to come. Professional quarrels and jealousies persisted especially in relation to consultation. There was no central authority to hear complaints or keep the profession in order.

In 1792, Thomas Percival, physician at the Manchester Royal Infirmary, at the request of the staff drew up a code of laws – later enlarged and called *Medical Ethics* (published 1803) – to set professional standards at that institution. It was a practical guide in a concrete situation to solve specific problems.[11] Its appeal was widespread for it was full of commonsense and generous wisdom telling a doctor exactly how to work with his colleagues and how best to serve the particular needs of the patient. Percival was himself a model of what he advised for others. From this book other codes were developed in the nineteenth century, particularly in the United States.

Early Scientific Medicine

The nineteenth century saw the dawn of scientific medicine, the foundations of which had been laid in the previous hundred years by such men as John Hunter. In his often quoted remark to Edward Jenner (the originator of vaccination), 'Why think? Why not try the experiment?', Hunter was stating a basic principle upon which experimental Medicine (the name given to physiology by Claude Bernard) was founded. It is significant that two great Frenchmen, Descartes and Bernard, both stepped aside from the path of scientific research in order to survey the principles upon which research should be conducted. Descartes in his 'Discours de la Méthode' (1637) had laid the foundations of the modern scientific method 'Pour atteindre à la vérité,' he wrote, 'il faut une foie dans sa vie se défaire de toutes les opinions que l'on a reçues et réconstruire de nouveau et dès la fondement, tous les systèmes des connaissances'. For Descartes the body was 'a machine made by the hand of God: incomparably better than any machine of human invention'. Man, in addition to possessing a body, however, was endowed with a mind which acted upon the body, and which could be demonstrated to exist by conscious thought: 'cogito, ergo sum'. 'Except our own thoughts, there is absolutely nothing in our power', wrote Descartes.

Claude Bernard re-inforced Descartes' view that there was no place in experimental medicine for doctrines or systems. 'Systems' he wrote, 'do not exist in nature but only in men's minds. . . . What we know may interfere with our learning what we do not know'.[12] The true scientist, according to Bernard, had no fixed starting point. He observed the facts of nature, from these facts he framed a hypothesis, and he next designed experiments to test the validity of his hypothesis. Imagination, though essential before and after experiment, had no place during the experiment, and should be shed, like one's overcoat, on entering the laboratory, only to be put on again on leaving. It was vital to preserve 'the independence and freedom of mind so essential to the progress of humanity'.

The firm establishment of morbid anatomy (Rokitanski and Virchow), the birth of bacteriology (Pasteur), the discovery of anaesthetics (Morton and Simpson), the advent of antiseptic surgery (Lister), the creation of the nursing profession (Florence Nightingale), the progress of public health, the discovery of X-rays, radium and vitamins, were all nineteenth-century advances bearing witness to the effectiveness of the scientific method.

Medical reform was in the air in the early nineteenth century but it was Charles Hastings, founder of the Provincial Medical and Surgical Association, 1832, (later to become the British Medical Association) who first began to give the idea a definite shape. The promotion of medical ethics was implied in the written objectives of the Association, particularly in the promotion of harmony and effective communication among members. The passing of the Medical Act in 1858 was largely promoted by the BMA.[13] At last, after many years of wrangling, and of ineffective local laws, the General Medical Council was empowered to control medical practice throughout the United Kingdom by limiting the right to practise to those whose names were enrolled in the Medical Register. Here, for the first time, doctors with their particular ethical standards and increasing scientific understanding became properly organized as a profession (see p. 19).

The Challenge of the Present

In the present century, we have seen the rise of specialization, the discovery of insulin and antibiotics, the invention of 'life support systems', the advent of tissue and organ transplantation, the widespread use of hormone therapy, to name but a few milestones in the path of medical progress, a path that appears to unroll before us at an ever increasing pace. Reflecting upon our medical heritage Sir William Osler wrote,[14] 'We may indeed be justly proud of our apostolic succession. Schools and systems have flourished and gone. . . . The Philosophies of one age have become the absurdities of the next, and the foolishness of yesterday has become the wisdom of tomorrow; through long ages which were slowly learning what we are hurrying to forget, amid all the changes and chances of twenty-five centuries, the profession has never lacked men who have lived up to the Greek ideals'.

During the golden ages of Greek and Renaissance Medicine, technical and theoretical advance went hand in hand with a deep concern for standards of practice (medical and ethical). The challenge of the present age of rapid and exciting technical advance is to remember that it is man and not the machine that ultimately matters. If we are to remain the masters of our technology and not become its slaves, we must never forget the patient is the middle of the apparatus that so often surrounds him. 'The more we know how to do things', wrote Sir Theodore Fox,[15] 'the more we shall need to know just what we really want to do. . . . We shall have to learn to refrain from doing things merely because we know how to do them'. If technical advance is not matched by an equal advance in ethical understanding and a maintenance of standards then the hospital becomes 'a life-saving chamber of horrors', and the doctor's surgery a pharmaceutical supermarket. Ethics must keep pace with science.

But if scientific medicine challenges the doctor to retain, above all, his humanity and common sense, the profession itself is threatened from a different direction by the growth of bureaucratic control over its affairs. For example, it is now being questioned in some circles whether the very existence of a self-governing profession is desirable. Whereas hitherto a doctor's conscience, his self-criticism and constant group assessment have served well to maintain his standards of patient care, the current suggestion (perhaps partly to curb overspending) is that public courts of enquiry or the investigations of the ombudsman would serve the public better to keep the doctor on his toes.

The notion behind such thinking is that everyone, including professional people, must be accountable to some superior officer, to corporate control and ultimately to the omnicompetent State. No one can be trusted; everyone must be watched. It is profoundly to be hoped these ideas are not put into practice. The best safeguard of the patient's interests is an independent well trained medical profession with high ethical standards. But how is the profession controlled at the present time?

The Profession's Ethics

With our increasing scientific understanding of the human body and increasing power over individual lives medical practitioners will always need guidance on what they ought and ought not to do. There are areas of difficult decision regarding the life and death of an individual. The diagnosis and treatment of disease may restrict patient freedom – how free should he be? The prevention of disease concerns society as a whole – what rules can be enforced? A fair distribution of national wealth is essential, but cost of medical care is increasing; how shall we decide where our limited resources are used?

Broadly speaking a doctor receives help on how to conduct his work from four sources, the law of the land, accepted professional standards, current philosophical ideas and religion.

The Law

Every doctor has a duty to obey the law of the land in the same way as every other citizen and he has to keep within it. Like any other person he is liable to be prosecuted and charged under the civil or criminal law if he is convicted of, say, assault, libel, negligence or particular motoring offences.

Secondly, in his work as a doctor there are specific laws which he has to observe in relation to such matters as prescription of dangerous drugs, the termination of a pregnancy, obtaining consent for an operation or conducting research on animals or humans.

Thirdly, the General Medical Council (GMC) was set up to determine who shall and who shall not practise medicine. The purpose was the protection of the public from unscrupulous and ill-qualified doctors. In order to achieve this the GMC was entrusted with the formation and maintainance of a Medical Register which is published annually; it contains the names of those who hold reputable qualifications as laid down in the Act.

Those whose names are on the Medical Registers are required to have attained a sufficiently high standard of education. Thus the Council has medical education constantly under review to ensure that doctors are well qualified to do their work in the light of modern knowledge. In the second place doctors are expected not to fall below those ethical standards which are consistent with the practice of good medicine. This ethical aspect of the Council's duties only evolved slowly over the years.

Initially the Council paid little attention to disciplinary matters but towards the end of the nineteenth century a change occurred. Any doctor acting in a way which could be construed as being dishonourable or disgraceful by his professional colleagues, who were in 'good repute and competency', could be considered guilty of infamous conduct. He could then be summoned before the Disciplinary Committee of the Council to answer charges laid before him. Two points should be noted: first that it was a judgment by his peers and secondly the definition of misconduct was a broad one. A doctor who came before the Committee was, if found guilty, liable to be warned, censured or perhaps have his name erased from the Register. This latter, in effect, deprived him of the right to practise.

What kind of offences came to the notice of the Council? Most commonly those reported to it by the police, where a doctor had been convicted of a crime by the civil courts. There were also those brought directly to the Council by members of the public, but the great majority of these were of a more trivial nature. Between 1901 and 1955 277 doctors were struck off the Register but most of them were restored after a year or two. Considering the increase in the number of doctors in the country over this period the number convicted is not large. The offences most commonly involved were adultery, procuring abortion, misuse of alcohol or drugs and advertising.

During the present century the Council has issued a 'Warning Notice' to a doctor when he registers to show him the kind of offences which have led to disciplinary action. Such matters as lax certification, covering (supporting an unqualified person to carry out treatment), advertising and disparagement of other practitioners are included.

It will be noted that rigid laws or rules are not laid down to govern a doctor's conduct. He has always been expected to have high moral standards precisely because his work is involved with the intimacies of human life and the sharing of human distress and because his power for good or evil is very great. Overall there is no doubt that the work of the General Medical Council has been of great benefit in sustaining the profession's reputation high in public esteem.*

The law thus both clarifies and circumscribes the field of action in which the doctor works. It is established by parliament for the good of the common people. Sir Thomas More once said 'the law is not a light for you or any man to see by; the law is not an instrument of any kind. The law is a causeway upon which, so long as he keeps to it a citizen may walk safely'. The doctor is a particular kind of citizen with special powers in his hands but he too has a causeway on which he may walk without fear in the service of his patients provided that he tries to be well informed and do what is right.

Accepted Professional Standards

It is of the nature of a profession to set its own standards of competence and continually keep them under review.

The Hippocratic Oath[16] whose main principles were outlined above, is by far the most famous code of conduct relating to the Medical Profession. It is timeless. One of its first recorded uses in Europe was at the University of Montpellier (founded 1181) where it was a form of promise made on graduating in Medicine. Many universities since, in Europe and the English-speaking world, have adopted the Oath – or a modification of it – as the ethical ideal for doctors.[17] In the last thirty years or so it has been questioned by some who insist that it has no relevance to modern medicine; it is ridiculed by not a few. Nevertheless, it is often given tacit support today and a recent Minister of Health could still taunt the profession with having renounced its Hippocratic Oath when, in the face of severe provocation, it threatened to reduce its services to the public. The Oath needs to be re-examined but its principles cannot be replaced or bettered.

Why was it that the Oath received such respect in Western Christendom over such a long time? Presumably because its main state-

* The more recent developments in the role of the General Medical Council are considered in chapter 3.

ments are broadly in accord with Christian ethics. It emphasizes the preservation and extension of such knowledge as will benefit humanity, a refusal to do harm or destroy life, a respect for the confidences of others and the maintenance of high standards of personal integrity. Such matters are largely beyond the scope of law and can only be achieved from within the Profession. The General Medical Council with its statutory powers, may be able to pick up those who stray too far off the highway, but it cannot dictate (nor has it ever attempted to) how doctors think and work.

Many attempts have been made in recent years to update Hippocrates. A Christian version was adopted in the early Church avoiding any invocation to Apollo or praise for the teacher and the clause which prohibits surgery (lithotomy) was dropped. With the rapid growth of medical science in recent years and the changing attitudes in society to human life and human need many new medical codes have been produced.

The Declaration of Geneva[18] was adopted by the World Health Organization in Geneva in 1948. In the next year, 1949, the general assembly of the World Medical Association adopted its own Code of Medical Ethics. The former retains the form of the Hippocratic Oath expressing it, so far as is possible, in modern language. The latter is a complete restatement of a doctor's duties covering more widely his relations with his patients. Both the Declaration and the Code owe much to the horror which was aroused by the activities of a small number of German doctors during World War II. In addition, there was a growing awareness of the power of medical science and the rights of individuals in the face of unjust oppression.

Other statements[19] have been made as a result of specific demands because of the growing effectiveness of medical treatment. *The Helsinki Declaration* (1964) gave recommendations to guide doctors in clinical research. *The Declaration of Sydney* (1968) discusses the timing of death and what is to be done if organ transplantation is contemplated. *The Declaration of Oslo* (1970) was a Statement on Therapeutic Abortion, while *The Declaration of Tokyo* (1975) guides doctors in their attitudes to torture and other cruel, inhuman or degrading treatment or punishment in relation to detention or imprisonment. Each of these was formulated at meetings of the World Medical Association.

All such post-war declarations serve to show how rapidly social life in the world is changing and how pervasive is the influence of modern medical science. The need for the profession to maintain high ethical standards is more than ever of vital importance.

General Philosophic Ethics

The laws of a nation define and classify moral values for ordinary men and women with regard to issues of life and death, human rights and human relationship. The ethical codes of the medical profession do the same for the doctor with his special responsibilities. Law reflects the moral consensus of the people; if it ceases to do so it needs to be changed. Many new laws have recently been passed because attitudes in Western Society have been changing.

What changes the moral attitudes of a people? The answer is the decline of a religion which no longer commands whole-hearted support, the introduction of new and contrary religions or different systems of thought and a general loss of respect for law and its sanctions as a proper means of maintaining order in society.

Mention has been made (see pp. 6–7) of some of the modern systems of thought which have particularly influenced attitudes to life in the past century – humanism, utilitarianism, existentialism – but many others could doubtless be described. What, perhaps, most affects the doctor now in his decision-making is 'situational ethics'. This simply means that when faced with an ethical dilemma in a clinical context the decision about what ought to be done is made not from laws or rules previously worked out as appropriate but from the situation as it presents itself there and then. In other words, a study of the situation itself will, it is thought, provide the right answer. In practice this may simply mean what the patient happens to want at the time.

Such an approach to problems puts the emphasis on the sympathy and spontaneity of the doctor and implies that he will find the right solution by intuition. But, whereas compassion is essential and a rigid conformity to rules can, on occasions, be cruel or damaging to a patient's best interest, situational ethics overlooks the fact that what we decide to do is often conditioned by the popular passing philosophy of the day or is influenced by the latest fad or fancy which has impressed us – or the patient. We can easily argue ourselves into making a wrongful decision appear praiseworthy. Some rules of what constitutes right and wrong for the individual, and what is best in the interests of society, must form the basis of ethical judgment, otherwise compassion becomes the sole arbiter for action and such a subjective quality cannot provide the justice which is the prime necessity in a stable community.

Religion

Many different religious views find expression in British society today. This may be true in the sense that we now have people of many other faiths living among us – Hindus, Sikhs, Muslims and perhaps a small sprinkling of Buddhists. But the influence of these groups on the nation's beliefs remains negligible even though their numbers have reached over two million. By no means all members of the coloured races among us adhere to these other faiths.

What is much more important is the all-pervasive 'non-religion' of the age. Very commonly now we set up man as the arbiter of his own destiny who then tries to find within himself the meaning and purpose of his own existence. No enduring ethical system can be derived from such ideas. Yet the media of communication, the television and the press, which so effectively reach men's minds and condition them to moral attitudes, are dominated by this secular outlook.

The Judaeo-Christian basis of Western civilization cannot easily be deposed nor do the many disruptive alternatives currently on offer commend themselves as possible long-term solutions. The medical profession, as it moves forwards into the exciting possibilities ahead needs to be mindful of what best serves both the individual patient and the community as a whole by holding fast to the well-tested truths of our Christian heritage and by remembering that the most important ethical values relating to human life are timeless and enduring.[20]

References

1. Johns, C. H. W. (Trans.) (1905) *The Oldest Code of Laws in the World*. Edinburgh.
2. von Klein, C. H. (1905) The Medical features of the Eber's papyrus. *Journal of the American Medical Association*. **45**, 26.
3. Nittis, S. (1942) Hippocratic ethics and present-day trends in medicine. *Bulletin of the History of Medicine*. **12**, 336.
4. Guthrie, D. (1945) *A History of Medicine*. London, Nelson, p. 82.
5. Corner, G. W. (1937) The Rise of Medicine at Salerno in the Twelfth Century, in *Lectures on the History of Medicine*. Mayo Foundation, p. 271.
6. Guthrie, D. *op. cit.* p. 103.
7. Richardson, Sir B. W. (1896) *Disciples of Aesculapius* (Francis Bacon) vol. 1. p. 402.
8. Richardson, Sir B. W. (1896) *op cit.* vol. **2**, p. 656.
9. Osler, Sir W. (1908) *An Alabama Student*.
10. King, Lester, S. (1958) *The Medical World of the Eighteenth Century*. University of Chicago Press.
11. King, L. S. *op cit.* p. 254.
12. Bernard, C. (1865) *An Introduction to the Study of Experimental Medicine*. Trans. H. C. Greene (1927). New York.
13. Little, E. M. *History of the British Medical Association 1832–1932*. London, BMA.
14. Osler, Sir W. (1904) *Aequanimitas and other Addresses*.
15. Fox, Sir T. (1960) *Lancet*, **2**, 801.
16. Recorded in full in the Appendix, p. 190.
17. Dr. Donald J. Guthrie, the medical historian, writes a fascinating chapter on the Hippocratic Oath in Davidson, M. (1957) *Medical Ethics*. London, Lloyd-Luke.
18. See appendix, p. 192.
19. See appendix for full texts of Declarations.
20. A modern Christian Affirmation on Medical Ethics is in the Appendix, p. 199.

Further Reading

BMA. (1974) *Medical Ethics*. London, British Medical Association.

Carr-Saunders, A. M. & Wilson, P. A. (1964) *The Professions*. London, Frank Cass.

Guthrie, D. (1945) *A History of Medicine*. London, Nelson.

Medical History and Medical Care (1971) *A Symposium of Perspectives*. London, Oxford University Press.

Poynter, F. N. L. (1961) *The Evolution of Medical Practice in Britain*. London, Pitman Medical.

Poynter, F. N. L. (1964) *The Evolution of Hospitals in Britain*. London, Pitman Medical.

Poynter, F. N. L. (1966) *The Evolution of Medical Education in Britain*. London, Pitman Medical.

Singer, C. & Underwood, E. A. (1962) *A Short History of Medicine*. London, Oxford University Press.

Taylor, J. Leahy (1970) *The Doctor and the Law*. London, Pitman Medical.

3

The Doctor's Freedom under Authority
David Warren

Medical practitioners have traditionally been accorded considerable liberty in their professional work, and often appeal to the right to 'clinical freedom' when outside restraints threaten to control their medical practice. While such an appeal might be a useful, if somewhat emotional, defence against unwelcome outside interference, it belies the fact that the work of doctors is already regulated in several ways. First, many aspects of the work of medical practitioners are governed by the law. When a doctor signs a prescription for drugs or a death certificate he must act within the regulations provided by law. If he physically examines or carries out an operation on a patient he must first obtain consent or he may find himself accused of assault and defending a claim for damages. The law operates both to protect the doctor in the exercise of his privileges, and to protect the public from the small number of doctors who might abuse their privileges, and the trust which they are normally accorded by their patients.

Second, hospital doctors are under contract to perform specified duties, and they are answerable to their employing authority if these duties are neglected. The employment of a hospital doctor may be terminated if he fails to comply with his contractual obligations. The Family Practitioner Committee within each Health Authority is responsible for the provision of general medical services, and may investigate many aspects of a general practitioner's work.

Third, the personal and professional conduct of doctors is governed by rules, mostly unwritten, which determine what is an acceptable standard of behaviour. These rules may be influenced by moral standards in the community at large and modified by legislation, but what they are and when they have been infringed, is determined by the consensus of the profession, and learnt by example. A doctor is ultimately accountable to his colleagues on the disciplinary committee of the General Medical Council if his personal and professional conduct falls below the accepted standard. The final arbiter of a doctor's conduct is his conscience, influenced in turn by his personal ethical code. The high level of personal responsibility which most doctors develop towards their patients early in their professional lives ensures that very few are ever called to account to their colleagues or the courts for their conduct.

The boundaries of the clinical freedom which a doctor enjoys are therefore hedged around by authority in various guises. His contractual obligations to his employer, his duty to obey the law of the land, his accountability to the GMC and his personal ethical standards

25

have been well recognized regulators of professional conduct for many years but within these constraints the doctor has been free to choose whether and how a patient should be treated. Recently several developments have restricted the freedom of the doctor to treat his patient in the way that he believes to be in accord with the best current treatment and in the most immediate interest of that patient. Legislation on social security benefits, abortion and homosexuality, and the practice of sterilization and artificial insemination have directly influenced the nature of the doctor-patient relationship. Patients are increasingly demanding that non-therapeutic procedures should be carried out upon them by medical practitioners. Changes in the standards of morality within the community produce conflicts in the minds of doctors whose personal standards are not changing at the same rate. Severe budgetary limitations within the National Health Service have further restricted the freedom of the doctor to choose the best treatment for his patient if that treatment is relatively expensive.

Reform of the General Medical Council

The principal functions of the General Medical Council, described in more detail in Chapter 2, include protection of the public by keeping a register of qualified medical practitioners and regulation of teaching standards. Discontent about the function of the General Medical Council was brought to a head by protests at the introduction of an annual retention fee payable by all practitioners intending to remain on the register. A Committee of Inquiry was subsequently set up under Sir Alec Merrison and reported in 1975. Doctors welcomed the proposed increase in the number and proportion of directly elected professional members (54 out of a total of 96) to a reconstituted body with wider functions in the field of specialist registration and the control of physically and mentally sick doctors. In addition, since through his place on the register the doctor gains public recognition of his professional competence, it was logical to give him a greater influence in the one body responsible for standards of training and conditions of registration. This increased freedom of action within the body responsible for regulating the profession carries with it greatly increased proposed authority of the Council over doctors whose competence to practise is reduced by ill-health. These two least contentious sections of the Merrison report were the subject of a Bill given its second reading in the House of Lords at the end of 1977. Other proposals for tighter control of the registration of overseas doctors and for a system of specialist registration are to be welcomed in principle since they are designed to protect and maintain high standards of medical practice. Of great concern is the fear that their implementation may limit the freedom of action of those currently on the medical register. Fortunately acceptance of proposals for increasing the number of doctors on the Council provides some assurance that the interests of currently registered doctors will be protected.

Much resentment has centred around the function of the General Medical Council as judge of the *mis*conduct of doctors, and the proposed change in emphasis towards a role as adviser in the field of professional conduct will be welcomed by all doctors. Thus the new General Medical Council, to which all qualified medical practitioners in the United Kingdom must pay an annual retention fee, will increase the freedom and influence of doctors within the community, while maintaining its own authority in the fields of registration and competence to practise. It is too early to know how well the balance will be struck.

Clinical Standards

'Audit' is a new word in the medical vocabulary, and in this context it means the development of an objective way of evaluating the quality of medical care provided by doctors. When applied to the administrative side of the National Health Service it is concerned with the efficient use of available resources, and as such is now an accepted part of the function of administrators at all levels. In the process of establishing that administrators have the right to make such assessments many senior hospital doctors have had to relinquish beds, clinics or research space in the interest of the health district as seen through administrative eyes. This process has been painful to many who cherish older concepts of the autonomy of the hospital consultant, and who failed to recognize the weakness of such concepts when physical and financial resources are limited. If the doctors who so resent 'administrative interference' were equally willing to become administrators themselves, and sit on the District Management Team, then their need to submit to authority could be tempered by their freedom to influence the direction and force of the Management Team's decisions. Audit in the form of assessment of the quality of health care in the United Kingdom has proved more difficult, though several attempts have been made in the United States. In 1970 the American Medical Association proposed the initiation of 'peer review organisations', and in 1973 the Joint Council on Accreditation of Hospitals insisted that medical audit should be set up in every hospital as a condition of accreditation. Since accreditation is essential to gain reimbursement from insurance companies and the government, the hospitals had little choice but to initiate medical audit. In 1974 medical audit became law with the setting up of the Professional Standards Review Organization (PSRO) designed to ensure the quality and duration of medical care provided under Medicaid and Medicare.

Such schemes sound attractive to the civil servant, the hospital administrator and the taxpayer who provide the resources but few will in practice be competent to measure standards of care. It is one thing to compare the cost incurred by two physicians in investigating a new hypertensive patient, but quite another to measure the quality of care meted out to the patient in the context of his illness, his family and his employment. It might be easy to examine a specialist's factual knowledge, and if necessary, re-educate him, but medical care implies far more than the demonstration of factual knowledge. Medical audit remains a concept which shows no signs of being attainable in a formal sense, and in the United States it carries undertones of sanctions against doctors with consequent limitation of their freedom to practise. Thus doctors will tend to practise 'defensive' medicine, with the primary object of avoiding blame rather than improving the quality of patient care. Such medical practice, with its emphasis on exploring every conceivable avenue of investigation of a patient in order to avoid an action for negligence, greatly increases the cost of medical care, the antithesis of the stated objectives of medical audit.

American style medical audit has few proponents in the United Kingdom where many believe that informed, responsible clinical freedom should be fostered. This implies an obligation on all doctors to contribute to and profit from collective knowledge, and to use it in a way which takes account of social and financial pressures. Thus all health districts provide continuing education courses for general practitioners, with financial inducements to the doctors and their teachers. Doctors in both hospital and general practice evolve methods for peer review based on case conferences or medical records. Hospital consultants are entitled to use up to 30 days in any 3-year period for attendance at conferences and training courses – with expenses paid. These processes of medical audit depend upon the mutual consent of the doctors caring for patients, not upon outside interference or threat of sanctions, and are in the best traditions of responsible professional practice. They imply willingness to change and re-education of those doctors whose parrot cries of 'clinical freedom' deafen their ears to improvements in medical care. More recently restriction of resources has added another dimension to medical audit, and idealism in medical decision-making must be tempered by awareness of financial limitations. Such a system of medical audit retains the clinical freedom of the doctor in his day to day relationship with his patients but subject to the authority of his peers.

Competence to Practise

No satisfactory system has yet been devised for the recognition of doctors who are unfit to practise through physical or mental illness. (see p. 175). This problem has been highlighted by the Merrison Report, and legislation to set up a Health Committee within the reconstituted General Medical Council is now progressing. If such doctors can be identified then the public is protected from incompetent medical care, and the normally high standards of the profession are maintained. In addition doctors who demonstrate incompetence by personal or professional negligence can be dealt with through the courts or the disciplinary processes of the General Medical Council.

The need for a formal mechanism for dealing with the sick doctor stems from the misplaced loyalty of his colleagues, who will either ignore his disability, whether it be deafness or alcoholism, or isolate him as a non-functioning member of the medical team. Neither course of action helps the doctor in question and to overcome this a formal procedure has been developed within the hospital service whereby a member of staff can inform one of three senior colleagues (the 'three wise men') who may make enquiries and if necessary report to the employing authority. No such formal procedure exists in general practice, and it remains to be seen how the 'three wise men' system becomes integrated with the General Medical Council health committee.

The Health Service Commissioner or ombudsman was first appointed in 1973 to look into administrative failures, delays, inadequate facilities or inadequate accommodation within the National Health Service. He cannot at present deal with the question of clinical competence, though the Health Councils have recently tried to institute procedures for dealing with complaints about clinical judgments of doctors. Such outside interference with the professional judgment of doctors poses the same threat of sanctions as American style medical audit, and would almost certainly lead to the practice of defensive medicine with all its disadvantages to the patient and the community.

Accountability

The public is protected by the generally high level of sensitivity among doctors in matters of professional conduct. The medical students or newly qualified doctor develops his own standards of professional conduct by observation of his senior colleagues, and at all levels within the profession the behaviour of a doctor is subject to the scrutiny of his senior and junior colleagues. Acceptable standards of professional conduct are learned by example rather than precept. Most doctors find that such a system works well in practice, though the 'unwritten rules' already referred to make assessment of individual doctors' professional standards almost impossible for a lay person except by reference to the standards within the profession as a whole. Where difficult problems arise, doctors are normally able to obtain the advice of their colleagues or their Medical Defence Society. In spite of these pressures within the profession to conform to an acceptable pattern of behaviour, errors are still made. Many of these result from the negligence or carelessness of the doctor, especially from his failure to visit, examine or treat a patient. Other complaints result from failure to observe professional secrecy, the conduct of wrong operations, intoxication of the doctor by alcohol or drugs and defamation of patients or colleagues.

The Department of Health has made clear to the hospital authorities that 'all patients should be provided before admission with a leaflet giving details of the person to whom written complaints and suggestions are to be made'. Minor complaints made orally are often dealt with to the complainant's satisfaction by the medical or nursing staff to whom they were initially made and it should be unnecessary to refer them to a senior member of the hospital administrative staff.

Family practitioner services are administered by Family Practitioner Committees and each of these committees appoints Service Committees which carry out investigations into complaints made by a patient or by another person on his behalf. Several courses of action are open to the Family Practitioner Committee if a doctor is found to be in breach of his terms of service. No action may be taken where the breach is trivial; a warning may be given to the doctor; the complainant's expenses may be withheld from the doctor's salary; or a larger sum may be withheld from the practitioner's remuneration. Excessive prescribing by doctors, record keeping, certification of patients for social security payment and complaints made by one doctor against another may also be investigated.

It can therefore be seen that doctors in general practice and in the hospital service may be called to account at many levels. They may be called to answer for their personal or professional conduct, but it is important to note that when professional conduct is in question, the doctor is answerable to his professional colleagues. This is as true of the General Medical Council as of the Service Committee investigating a complaint of a professional nature against a general medical practitioner. The rules of conduct governing the profession (whether written or unwritten) are laid down by its members, and it is to be hoped that the principle of accountability within the medical profession will be maintained. The Merrison Report certainly expects this to continue to be the case following any reorganization of the General Medical Council. It will be a tragic reflection on the integrity of the medical profession if legislation ever becomes necessary to regulate from outside the professional conduct of doctors.

Recent Legislation and the Doctor's Freedom

The cherished concept of 'clinical freedom' referred to at the beginning of this chapter is largely illusory. A doctor's personal integrity and ethical code must be of a very high order if his professional practice is to be uninfluenced by the many forces which combine to bend his mind and actions to the wishes of others. Glossy brochures, attractively designed and carefully and persuasively worded arrive on his doormat from pharmaceutical companies each day. The many apparently valuable therapeutic effects claimed for a new drug disappear when critical reading of the wording often shows it to be almost meaningless advertising jargon. There have been remarkable but irrational changes in the prescribing habits of doctors as the result of clever marketing of new drugs (see p. 120).

Certification   Equally pernicious in the restriction of a doctor's freedom is the effect of public opinion expressed through the personal demands of his patient for particular services. Doctors in general medical practice sign certificates of incapacity to work every day. Most of these are statutory forms used by the patient to apply for social security benefits. The doctor is required to examine the patient and to be of the opinion that he is unable to work for a stated period. Family doctors have the advantage of knowing their patients and especially those with chronic or serious illnesses and can sign statutory certificates of this nature without hesitation.

Much more difficulty is experienced when the patient presents with vague complaints, no significant physical findings and a request for 'a week or two on the club'. Any hesitation on the doctor's part may provoke indignant protests from the patient that he is entitled to social security benefits because of his weekly payments. Prolonged argument with such a patient would only produce administrative chaos in a busy surgery. Since the doctor is unable to prove that the patient does not have an illness, the advantage clearly lies with the patient and he may well present himself to another partner in the same practice if met with a refusal from the first doctor.

Hospital doctors also find their professional judgment about a patient compromised by those who, for various reasons, present themselves for admission at emergency departments with symptoms which are claimed to be severe and which the doctor cannot disprove. Although some such patients are seeking satisfaction of their drug addiction, this is not always the case, and there are some who spend many weeks each year in hospital without significant organic disease being discovered. These examples of manipulation of doctors by patients are well known and it is difficult to see an easy solution to the ethical problems raised. Quite apart from the professional aspect of such cases, they lead doctors to compromise their role as stewards of very large sums of public money. It is unlikely that a free comprehensive health-care service and the provision of financial benefits to all those genuinely entitled to them can be administered without abuse. It follows that most doctors will at some time find their professional judgment compromised in their efforts to ensure that proper care is received by all who are entitled to it.

Termination of Pregnancy   The abuses discussed above are the indirect result of the legislation by which the health-care and social security benefits are administered. There is increasing pressure within society for legislation which will directly affect the nature of medical practice. The 1967 Abortion Act is the outstanding example of such legislation.

The Abortion Act (1967) did not legalize abortion, which remains a criminal offence (see p. 64). It created exceptions by providing that an offence is not committed when pregnancy is terminated under certain circumstances. Most important to the present discussion is the provision that pregnancy may be terminated if its continuance would involve risk to the life or health of the pregnant woman greater than if the pregnancy was terminated. The effect of this Act on the practice of general medical practitioners, obstetricians and gynaecologists has been greater than the legislators could possibly have envisaged. The intention of the Act was not to provide for abortion on demand since no gynaecologist was to be under obligation to terminate a pregnancy if, in his clinical opinion, the operation was not indicated. However, the effect of the legislation in contrast to its intention has been to permit such wide interpretation of the terms 'physical or mental health of the mother' that women who wish to have their pregnancy terminated have no difficulty in finding doctors willing to sign the official forms. Although the Act does not allow abortion on social grounds, it is also apparent that trivial difficulties within a woman's social environment can be used to argue that to allow the pregnancy to continue might, in the future, damage the mother's mental or physical health.

Once a liberal interpretation of the Act is advocated and inplemented by a section of the medical profession, other doctors who favour an interpretation more in keeping with the spirit of the Act find themselves in an almost impossible position. The combination of loosely worded legislation, liberalization of public attitudes to abortion and the readiness of a section of the medical profession to interpret the law as widely as possible has effectively forced many doctors to practise a more liberal interpretation of the Act than their better judgment would sanction. It is still possible that this legislation will rebound on itself; increasing evidence of the long-term injurious effects of abortion on the health of a woman and any further children she may bear may force reconsideration of the assumption that in almost any socially inconvenient situation continuation of the pregnancy would involve risk to the life or health of the mother greater than if the pregnancy were terminated.

The Abortion Act is used here as an example of how society, by public pressure and legislation, may change the doctor-patient relationship. Legislation has increased the freedom of women to dispose of unwanted pregnancies, but has limited the freedom of their doctors to advise them in the light of all the clinical, social and ethical considerations surrounding their case.

Euthanasia   Euthanasia is likely to come before parliament again in the near future and no doubt another voluntary euthanasia Bill will include conditions thought necessary by the legislators to protect both the patients who might become the subjects of euthanasia and their doctors (see p. 101). In spite of all the safeguards that might be included, it might be only a short time after the passage of such a Bill before involuntary euthanasia became accepted, if not demanded, by the community as a means of disposing of congenitally deformed neonates or patients with senile dementia. A successful voluntary euthanasia Bill would comprise the practice of a much larger section of the profession than the Abortion Act and destroy the trust which at present characterizes the doctor-patient relationship.

The Abortion Act 1967 provides that 'no person shall be under any duty, whether by contract or any other statutory or legal requirement, to participate in any treatment authorized by this Act to which he has a conscientious objection' though the doctors' duty to 'participate in treatment which is necessary to save life or prevent grave permanent injury to the mental health of a pregnant woman' remains. Similar wording was used in the last, unsuccessful, Euthanasia Bill. In the context of the Abortion Act 1967 the provision for conscientious objection has ceased to have any meaning. A doctor who has such objections to carrying out abortions will find it virtually impossible to obtain a post of Consultant Obstetrician and Gynaecologist in Britain, and this state of affairs appears to enjoy the blessing of the Department of Health. Public pressure, expressed through legislation, has forced the medical profession to conform to a particular pattern of conduct, and as a result, effectively excluded from practice (as obstetricians and gynaecologists) those doctors who express conscientious objections.

Traditional roles have thus been reversed, and unless doctors recognize the way in which this one area of medical practice has become subject to the authority of public opinion they may find themselves unwittingly coerced through legislation into other far-reaching restrictions on their medical practice.

National Health Service Reorganization

The Department of Health stated in 1972 that 'The aims in reorganisation are, first that there should be a fully integrated Health Service in which every aspect of health care can be provided by members of the health care profession and second, that this care should be provided as far as possible locally and with due regard to the health needs of the community as a whole'. These aims were to be implemented by integration of general practitioner, hospital and public health services and more effective contributions by doctors to NHS decision-making. Co-ordination of health care within the framework of Area Health Authorities and Districts was also intended to correct disparities among regions and specialities, with redistribution of their resources where necessary.

The principal innovation as far as practising doctors were concerned was the establishment of District Management Teams, each with a consultant and general practitioner as members. These teams are concerned with the health needs of local populations of up to 300,000 and it was expected that they would be sensitive to local needs and priorities. With the establishment of District Management Teams senior hospital consultants have lost some traditional privileges. In one hospital known to the author the senior of 4–5 consultants on each medical unit used to be known as 'Consultant in Administrative Charge' and could exercise an authoritarian control over 'his' registrars and 'his' beds. This title has disappeared with NHS reorganization but not every consultant is willing to relinquish a registrar because the needs of the service require the post to be transferred elsewhere. Decision-making has become more cumbersome since certain members of staff, such as senior consultants and medical superintendents, have lost a large measure of their traditional personal authority. The consequent proliferation of committees has been a major source of irritation to members of the health service in clinical practice. Although individuals have clearly lost a measure of personal authority over their share of health service facilities, the general standard of health care in a community should be improved by the sharing of available resources as the result of consensus between representatives of different branches of the service. It is unfortunate that NHS reorganization has come at a time of economic decline, so that reallocation of resources in many cases means in practice the restriction of growth in some areas of the service. With improvement in the economic climate it is likely that the functions of the District Management Team will be seen in a more positive light. Reorganization has increased the freedom of the hospital doctor by giving him an administrative role but at the same time subjected him to the authority of his colleagues.

Since the administrative structure of the hospital service was clarified by reorganization it has become increasingly subject to pressures from the Health Service trades unions. The unions' principal concern is the interest of its members (not the hospital patient), therefore union pressures in the form of strikes or 'blacking' of private beds are compounding the disruption to the hospital services caused by financial restraint. Most doctors are surprisingly complacent about the actions of Health Service unions, but this indifference will only further diminish the patient as the principal objective of health-care, and the doctor as the decision-maker in respect of the patient who came to him for help.

Doctors and Industrial Action

During the last three years most doctors in clinical practice had to face seriously the question of withdrawal of labour for the first time. The principal issues, new contracts for hospital doctors, the phasing out of pay beds and proposals for reallocation of resources within the National Health Service, serve to maintain the present level of resentment among hospital doctors. Many hospital doctors have engaged in industrial action, though lack of unity within the profession has left the political effectiveness of this action open to doubt. That many patients have been seriously inconvenienced is not in doubt, and the news media have been quick to publicize a few cases where delay in hospital admission because of industrial action by doctors might have been responsible for the death of a patient.

A recent letter to the Lancet suggested that the 'administration would like to treat doctors as workers and expects them to behave like a profession'. It is just because doctors are both workers and members of a profession that industrial action raises serious ethical problems and the freedom of doctors to take strike action is questioned. As workers doctors receive remuneration from the state in return for their services. Many are members of trades unions such as the Medical Practitioners Union or the British Medical Association. In common with other groups of workers with high incomes they are very sensitive to the maintenance of their status, and the British Medical Association used the erosion of the relative status and income of doctors as one of the principal grounds for proposed industrial action in late 1974. As employees of the State doctors are not immune from changes in national priorities which might result in reconsideration of traditional income differentials between, say, doctors and coal miners.

Just as the ultimate sanction of an employer is dismissal from service, so the ultimate action of the employee against the employer is withdrawal of labour. Many doctors have come to regard the 'right to strike' in the same way as an engineering worker, ignoring the fundamentally different obligations. These differences arise from the traditional professional nature of medical practice, which puts the interest of the patient before the self-interest of the doctor. It is difficult to see how the patient could be sure of getting the best advice and treatment if this were not true. It is particularly so in the National Health Service where the doctor is not put under any obligation to his patients as the result of a personal financial transaction.

Three main courses of action have been proposed by doctors as a protest against the Department of Health. In some hospitals there has been complete withdrawal of labour by junior doctors for a limited period, such as 24 hours. Such action has not been a very effective protest because a significant number of doctors are not prepared to take this action in support of their more militant colleagues. Much greater support has been obtained for action to treat emergency cases only, though what constitutes an emergency is difficult to define. Many patients must be seen and examined by a doctor before the nature and severity of their illness can be determined. Lastly, many doctors see resignation from the National Health Service as the only honourable form of protest. This proposal includes provisions for doctors to be employed by hospitals through a medical employment agency. There are ethical objections to all of these courses of action.

Few doctors appear to have considered the practical implications of strike action. The British Medical Association has no funds with which to support doctors on strike and there can be few who would not find themselves under severe financial strain if their salary were withdrawn in response to industrial action. For this reason alone the threat of strike action is unlikely to force the Government into relaxing its wage policy for doctors.

There is nothing in the doctor's professional code to permit a distinction between his obligations to urgent and non-urgent clinical problems. His primary obligation is to the patient, whether he presents with a hernia of ten years duration or is in shock following a haemorrhage. Refusal to see the patient with a hernia may burden the doctor's conscience less than if he refuses to resuscitate a man dying of haemorrhage, but this does not excuse the disregard of one of the most important principles of professional medical practice. In the author's view, no amount of dissatisfaction with the Government's policy can justify refusal to see patients. Because of these ethical constraints many doctors have felt that mass resignation is the only morally defensible course of action. While this may be a logical step for an individual doctor, the absence of alternative medical services means that mass resignation raises the same problems in relation to patients as strike action.

At the present time there is no truly representative body to negotiate the remuneration of doctors and few of them believe that the annual recommendations of the Review Body are independent of the Government. The increased militancy of doctors is probably here to stay and the first step in restoring confidence in the Department of Health depends on the establishment of a representative independent negotiating body. Because of the nature of medical professional practice the doctor does not have the freedom to withdraw from patient care. This does not prevent the profession from doing all in its power to bring to the attention of the Government the limitations of the service, and real injustices where they occur.

Further Reading

Hill, D. (1977) The General Medical Council: Frame of reference or arbiter of morals? *Journal of Medical Ethics*, 3, 110.

Koran, L. M. (1975) The reliability of clinical methods, date and judgements. *New England Journal of Medicine*, **293**, 642.
McNerney, W. J. (1976) The quandary of quality assessment. *New England Journal of Medicine*, **295**, 1505.

4

Problems Arising from Genetic Advances
Robert and Caroline Berry

Genetics is a new recruit to ethical discussion. There are two reasons for this. First, as diseases resulting from infection and malnutrition have in principle been brought under control, those dependent upon or affected by inherited factors have become both relatively and absolutely more important in western countries. For example, congenital malformations now cause about one quarter of neonatal deaths, whereas they accounted for less than two per cent at the turn of the century although their incidence has remained more or less constant. Second, our better understanding of gene action has now made possible the rational treatment of many inherited diseases – by the elimination of offending molecules from the diet (galactosaemia, phenylketonuria), replacement of defective gene products (haemophilia, diabetes mellitus), elimination of excessive accumulations of metabolites (Wilson's disease), or surgical treatment (multiple polyposis).

Genetic problems have, therefore, become much more obtrusive in medical practice. The incidence of genetic disease detectable at birth is about three per cent, while a further one per cent of the population is affected later in life (Table 4.1), so every doctor is likely to be faced with it at some stage. Such diseases give rise to ethical challenges different from those traditionally arising in clinical medicine because,

1. In most cases, the person who consults the doctor is not the patient but a normal relative, usually a parent or potential parent of an affected individual.
2. The advice offered may be the prevention of birth of an affected person, either by the parents agreeing to have no natural children of their own or by selective abortion following prenatal diagnosis of an abnormality.
3. Families and societies have a limited ability to cope with sickness. They may judge that they are better served by preventing the birth of certain children than by allowing their birth and then supporting them.
4. New biological techniques for controlling human reproduction raise spectres of Huxley's 'Brave New World'. These are largely problems of the future, but they already cause anxiety for some.

The problems arising from these points can be considered under four headings although in practice they overlap – genetic counselling, prenatal diagnosis and selective abortion, individual versus social good and genetic engineering.

38

Table 4.1 *Incidence of Genetic Disease in Man**

Type of Inheritance	Incidence per 1000 births	
Single gene effect		
Autosomal dominant	9.5	
Autosomal recessive	1.3	
Sex-linked recessive	0.4	
All single locus effects		11.2
Chromosome anomalies		
Trisomy-21	1.4	
Trisomy-13	0.1	
Trisomy-18	0.2	
Cri du chat	<0.1	
Klinefelter's syndrome, etc. } in males	1.7	
XYY syndrome	c.0.1	
XXX syndrome } in females	1.0	
Turner's syndrome	0.2	
Total clinical major chromosomal anomalies	5.4	
Congenital malformations	14.1	
Serious 'constitutional' disorders (diabetes mellitus, idiopathic epilepsy, schizophrenia, etc.)	14.8	

* From Berry, R. J. (1972) Genetical effects of radiation on populations. *Atomic Energy Review*, 10, 67–100.

Genetic Counselling

About 90% of those seeking help are couples who have already produced an abnormal child or know of one in their family. Increasingly, couples at risk for particular reasons, especially maternal age, are wanting guidance. The probability of the birth of an abnormal child is an entirely technical matter, but the circumstances in which counselling is sought tend to be emotive and, if badly handled, unnecessary distress may result. Furthermore, the counsel offered to a couple may itself involve them in moral problems.

Usually, parents can be given all available information and most of them appreciate being so informed, even when the outlook is bad. Practical problems may arise through their lack of understanding. For example, if a child with an inherited defect appears to be doing well, they may not appreciate the difficulties they will face coping with a later, more severe stage of the disease (as in muscular dystrophy) and consequently they will not realize the implications of having another affected child. Again, one parent may feel guilt or anger at causing an abnormality (such as transmitting a translocated chromosome), thereby causing marital disharmony or demands for sterilization. The responsibility of the counsellor, therefore, extends further than a mere recitation of the risks of having another affected child; often he will be asked what is the wisest decision to make. It may then be necessary to explain, in language appropriate to the couple concerned, the different consequences and possible courses of action, or even to give a personal opinion.[1]

There are six criteria that may be employed by parents in making a decision about future pregnancies:

1. The risk of producing an affected child.
2. The severity of the disorder. In some conditions death in early infancy may be virtually certain, and many parents are more willing to risk having such an infant than to face a protracted illness of many years duration.
3. The physical, emotional and economic impact on the family and on society.

   Less important are:

4. The availability of adequate medical management and of special educational and other facilities.
5. The predictability of the expression of the disorder involved.
6. And, possibly, the recognition that an individual who is genetically defective in one respect may be superior in others or may compensate by the development of other abilities or talents.

In practice the most important factors influencing parental decisions are the severity of the condition and the magnitude of the risk. The majority of couples given a risk of less than one in ten of their child's being affected opt for further pregnancies.[2] The high risk serious conditions are mainly recessively-inherited traits (cystic fibrosis, various inborn errors of metabolism) where each parent is heterozygous and together they have a one in four chance of producing an affected homozygote. Only a proportion of the relevant dominantly inherited conditions (such as Marfan's Syndrome) are seriously handicapping, but the children of such an affected individual have a one in two chance of being affected themselves. The options open to such couples – apart from childlessness – are adoption or artificial insemination by donor. For conditions where prenatal diagnosis is available, they may choose to proceed with a pregnancy and face the possibility of a therapeutic abortion if an abnormality is found (see below).

Family Studies

Sometimes the detection of an 'abnormality', such as a translocated chromosome in a congenitally abnormal infant, suggests that other members of the family of one parent should be investigated to see whether they too are at risk of having a similarly abnormal offspring. Where family relationships are good, this is no problem and the people concerned can be investigated and counselled appropriately. In some families, however, the parents may not want other members approached and the investigator is in the unfortunate position of knowing of people in need of advice – and indeed at risk – but feeling bound by his patient's desire for confidentiality.[3] At present, the doctor's prior duty appears to be to his patient, rather than to a relative who is only a hypothetical patient. This problem is discussed further in the section on the individual and society (p. 44).

If family studies can be carried out, the action to be taken depends on the nature of the condition under consideration. For example, in polyposis coli, which is a dominantly inherited condition associated with a high risk of death from carcinoma of the colon, relatives can be advised to submit themselves to investigation so that the condition can be detected and treatment considered before malignant change has occurred. Thus, affected relatives can safeguard themselves and their offspring from the effects of the gene. In Huntington's chorea the situation is entirely different. This degenerative condition of the central nervous system manifests itself only in middle age, by which time the patient will have unknowingly passed on the gene to some children and through them to grandchildren. At present, those at risk can only be warned that they may develop the disease in later life and that if they are found to carry the gene each child of theirs also has a 50-50 chance of being similarly affected. If carriers could be recognized in early life, those shown to be unaffected would be at liberty to procreate freely, while gene carriers would have to live with the knowledge that they would develop an extremely unpleasant incurable disease in middle age or earlier. If such a test becomes available the decision as to whether it should be used or not will have to be carefully assessed for each individual concerned. It is to be hoped that any advance in knowledge which makes detection possible will also result in progress towards treatment or specific prevention.

The advent of prenatal diagnosis has made family studies for conditions which can be detected in this way both more worthwhile and more acceptable. It is now possible to advise family members of their risks and at the same time offer them a means of avoiding such a risk.

Prenatal Diagnosis and Selective Abortion

The genetic constitution of an individual is determined at conception. Between a third and a half of all zygotes spontaneously abort, most of them in the first few weeks of pregnancy, approximately 40% of them because of an abnormal chromosome complement. Most of them are lost early (97% of Turner's syndrome and 65–70% of Down's syndrome have been aborted by the 18th week). It seems likely that a large proportion of those with central nervous system anomalies are also spontaneously aborted. Modern techniques can identify many of the abnormal fetuses which survive elimination in this way. Selective abortion is able to bring about further reduction in the incidence of certain diseases.

At present prenatal diagnosis requires amniocentesis to obtain amniotic fluid and fetal cells. These can be cultured for chromosome analysis and biochemical assays. Most open neural tube defects are detected by the level of alpha-fetoprotein in amniotic fluid. Ultrasound can also be used to help in diagnosis. The techniques of fetal blood sampling and fetoscopy are still in the early stages of development but, if they become established, they will allow the detection of an increasing number of fetal abnormalities during the second trimester in those at high risk.

Herein lie the ethical problems. Is it right to use abortion in order to reduce the incidence of a disease such as Down's syndrome where sufferers are apparently capable of a happy, albeit limited existence? Should selective abortion be used in the case of all abnormalities identified or only the more serious ones? Those who have a high regard for individual human life may consider the termination of pregnancy unacceptable. But even those prepared to tolerate selective termination have to take into consideration other factors than the degree of deformity, even when we can predict that accurately. For example is not the limited life of the child with Down's syndrome or the short life of one with spina bifida also a gift which God bestows? There are mothers who have gladly cared for their deformed baby during its short life and would not have had it otherwise.

It is possible to distinguish four situations:

a) Where a diagnosis of abnormality can be made with certainty and the implications for future life are foreseeable, for example, in Down's syndrome, in many biochemical disorders such as Tay-Sachs disease, and with large open spina bifida cases.

b) Where diagnosis is certain but the implications of it are uncertain. For example, the same sex chromosome abnormality may vary considerably in its expression in different individuals. Only a proportion have mental deficiency or illness but otherwise there is so little effect apparent that they are frequently not diagnosed at all. As chromosome staining and banding techniques improve it may be possible to forecast the severity of various diseases more precisely than at present, but it is more likely that the multitude of small variations (polymorphisms) that are now recognized will complicate the interpretation.[4] Similarly, developments in fetoscopy will lead to the recognition of minor defects which will create new ethical problems as to how much information to give the patient and the criteria for advising termination.

c) In some cases a definite diagnosis may not be possible, but a high risk of inherited disease may be present. For example, male children of a female known to be a carrier (i.e. heterozygous) for a sex-linked recessive condition (such as haemophilia or Duchenne's muscular dystrophy) have a 50% chance of being affected. Since the sex of fetuses can be determined, termination of pregnancy can be offered in the case of all males. This means that a normal fetus will be eliminated as often as an affected one. However, such action may be the only possible alternative to not having a family which is acceptable to a woman who has herself observed the suffering of a severely affected son or brother.

d) Fetuses may be indentified who will be normal, but carriers of undesirable traits. These include daughters of men suffering from a sex-linked recessive condition, such as haemophilia, and individuals with a translocated chromosome. The extreme situation in this group is a fetus of the 'wrong' sex for its parents. It is impossible to justify termination in such cases solely under the section of the Abortion Law which refers to fetal abnormality.

Most centres accept that a discussion leading to a commitment to abortion – or at least to consider abortion – should precede amniocentesis. It is claimed that prior knowledge of either disease or normality may relieve anxiety in a couple and prepare them for the child to be born,[5] but some patients are so anxious that even an amniocentesis may produce such emotional stress that they are unsuitable for investigation. Some women ask to be tested 'to be on the safe side', but unless there are specific grounds for believing that they might produce an abnormal child, the risk of amniocentesis – albeit slight – should be sufficient to persuade the doctor to advise her not to undergo the test.

Mothers known to be at risk of having an abnormal infant may refuse prenatal diagnosis on religious or conscientious grounds, or because any interference with a longed-for pregnancy is unacceptable. As prenatal diagnosis becomes more widely available, the attitude of society may become the over-riding factor. For example, will medical and other supporting facilities (including institutional care) continue to be freely available for those who decline prenatal diagnosis on the understanding that they will rear their possibly abnormal child themselves? Will the attitude of the general public, which at present is becoming more tolerant to those who have handicaps, harden to the view that 'they should never have been born'?

Prenatal diagnosis and selective abortion open up a new dimension in medical ethics, since they aim at the elimination of abnormal individuals rather than cure or palliation. Unless used with wisdom and awareness, it could become the thin end of a very long wedge causing major changes in attitudes towards life and disease.

Individual Versus Social Good

The main consideration of a couple faced with the possibility of producing an abnormal child are the problems that the abnormality may cause to the child and to themselves, but there are also the remedial, educational and financial difficulties which society faces with its abnormal members. Primitive societies can absorb a proportion of mentally or physically handicapped members, but this is increasingly expensive in money and manpower in modern urban communities. It has been estimated that life-long institutional care of, for example, a person with Down's syndrome, costs £150,000.

The situation is analogous to that which arose in the nineteenth century with the discovery of the methods of spread of infectious diseases when legislation was introduced solely to safeguard the public at large, rather than the affected person's household. Now that the rules of occurrence of genetically determined diseases are beginning to be understood, we need to ask what steps society might or should take to regulate them. There are three areas of possible concern – population screening, compulsion and confidentiality and genetic load.

Population Screening (see p. 85)

Hitherto, we have considered situations where a patient or his parents comes to a doctor asking for advice. Screening works in the opposite direction. A search is made by a third party for those at risk, warning them of the effects of the disease – personally or in their children – and what action, if any, they can take.

Such breaking into lives of others may do more harm than good. For example, a screening programme for sickle cell anaemia in the USA has been challenged by accusations of racialism, because the condition is much more common in blacks than whites. Consequently, it is important to appreciate what are the goals of screening.[6] They can be summarized as follows:

1. *The provision of benefits to individuals* by identifying disease when it is early and treatable (phenylketonuria, diabetes, or Wilson's disease, see p. 38).
2. *Identifying carriers of inherited diseases* in order to warn them of the risk to themselves or their children. Two groups are involved – those who carry a dominant gene with low penetrance, though they themselves show little evidence of the condition, and those who are heterozygous for recessive disorders. For the former, their children have a 1:2 risk of carrying the gene but an uncertain risk as to how severely affected they will be. The latter group include some relatively common diseases, such as Tay-Sachs disease in Ashkenazi Jews or sickle cell anaemia in people of African origin. It is this latter group which gives rise to most ethical problems.
3. *Research projects* even though they may be of little or no immediate benefit to those detected by the screening programme. Indeed, knowledge of variations detected in this way can often be embar-

rassing. For example, screening may lead to the identification of an XYY boy.[7] The 'abnormal' boy might then receive extra help and guidance, but there is a risk that he might suffer prejudice from a school-teacher, or law court on the grounds of being 'biologically abnormal'. Indeed, screening could lead to a false emphasis on 'normality', producing pressures for abortion, guilt on the part of parents refusing to participate and new attitudes to the genetically different.

4. *Reduction in the frequency of apparently deleterious alleles* (see section below on 'Genetical Engineering').

Problems in a Screening Programme The fact that a high proportion of the population has to be screened demands publicity and co-operation with the local community. Any form of compulsion is unacceptable in a 'free' society although the offering of inducements seems to be acceptable. Ideally, those shown to be at risk should be able to protect themselves by prenatal diagnosis and abortion, although this causes difficulties for those who conscientiously object to termination of pregnancy. For example, because Tay-Sachs disease in a fetus can be diagnosed prenatally, screening has been more acceptable and successful than for sickle cell disease, where prenatal diagnosis is only just becoming available and couples at risk are only offered sterilization.

An essential part of any screening programme is the ready availability of facilities for follow-up by fully trained genetic counsellors. They can provide easily understood explanations for those whose conditions have been detected with the aim of ensuring that individuals do not spend the rest of their lives under a misapprehension. An example of this occurred in the sickle cell screening programme in the USA where many heterozygotes believed themselves to be unhealthy and in some cases even lost their jobs because of misapprehension by employers.

In this country, the only recessive condition sufficiently common to warrant general population screening is cystic fibrosis. As yet, no reliable test is available for either the detection of heterozygotes or the prenatal diagnosis of homozygotes, but this may well change within the next few years.

At present under serious consideration – and the subject of a large scale pilot investigation – is the screening of all pregnant women by serum alpha-fetoprotein estimation with a view to detecting open spina bifida and anencephaly in the fetus. The logistic problems are formidable but not insurmountable. Ethical difficulties can also be foreseen, since for those to whom termination of pregnancy is unacceptable there must be an opportunity to opt out. Since a raised serum AFP is only suggestive of fetal abnormality an urgent amniocentesis has to be arranged for those women with raised serum levels and yet time must be found for careful explanation to both the patient and her husband if misunderstanding and unnecessary anxiety are to be avoided.

Compulsion and Confidentiality

Because of the way in which genetic disease is transmitted there is now popular interest in the identification of human traits judged to be undesirable (there is interest too in desirable traits relating to race and intelligence). The problem of compulsion and confidentiality is more acute with large scale surveys, where computers are used and many people have access to the results. For example, the police might demand access to the results of a screening programme and the discovery of abnormal sex chromosome complements (especially XYY males) could be used by those concerned with either the defence or prosecution of an alleged malefactor. Policies for such an event should be decided beforehand. Linked to the question of confidentiality is the reluctance of some to submit to genetic investigation. This may be due to a general fear of the findings or, sometimes, the exposure of sexual irregularity. If sterilization is proposed on genetic grounds, the question arises whether compulsion is ever justified. Fortunately, the good of the individual and family usually coincides with the course of action which is best for society. When contrary occasions arise, the wisest course of action seems to be tactful persuasion of the individual concerned, as at present any form of coercion in this emotive field tends to produce acute reaction and publicity. The problem of compulsory sterilization is by no means academic, since the current policy of treating retarded patients within the community rather than in institutions means that opportunities for pregnancy increase considerably. A woman with Down's syndrome has a 50-50 chance of having a similarly affected child, a figure that has been borne out by the few such pregnancies reported.

When there is a conflict of interest between the patient and society, the decision should possibly be referred to a panel with both lay and medical members. One difficulty is that a decision may be needed rapidly in the case of a pregnant patient. There is also the point that group decisions may be less human than that of an individual undertaking personal responsibility, and such a decision could well be less acceptable to the person concerned than that of a single physician.

In addition to the ethics of the procedures themselves, their cost must be considered. Techniques of investigation are expensive, and prenatal diagnosis is really only feasible in developed countries. Against this must be set the problem that the cost of caring for congenitally abnormal children is greater in societies where they cannot be easily absorbed into the community. In other words, the issues of both compulsion and confidentiality are to some extent culture-dependent, and need to be continually reviewed.

Genetic Load

A small, but probably increasing number of parents are concerned about the growing genetic burden as a result of the medical success in achieving survival of those with inherited defects and allowing the transmission of genes that would previously have resulted in sterility. In addition there is an increase of mutations induced by man-made agencies such as ionizing radiations and a range of new chemicals in the environment.*

The idea of a 'genetic load' dragging mankind to early extinction was put forward by Müller in 1950, and was wrong on two counts. Müller's prophecy was based on the assumption that family size was a biological constant, whereas we can (and do) adjust our conception rate in response to early genetic mortality. In addition, all mutation is not harmful, as was believed by Müller.

Most chromosomal anomalies are dominant lethals (i.e. their carriers do not hand them on), and the role of gene mutation in maintaining population variation is probably small. This is a technical question which cannot be argued here. It is only relevant in this context to point out that the vast majority of conditions with a genetic component are multifactorially determined, and selection would have to be very stringent to affect gene frequencies significantly. Indeed, the selective pressures acting on the human species may be as strong today as they ever were, albeit different in direction with the changes in our environment.[8] This does not affect the immediate medical and social problems of genetic disease – it merely confounds the ratiocinations of intellectuals.

Genetic Engineering

To many, the spectre of genetic control is of the stuff of science fiction. In fact, the fashionable term 'genetic engineering' conceals a number of activities relevant to practising doctors.

In 1869, Galton published his *Hereditary Genius* demonstrating the transmission of valuable social or manipulative skills in particular families. He followed this by advocating *eugenics*, a term he invented in 1883. This was a time of concern on one hand of genetic deterioration, and on the other the utilitarian ideal of progress. The obvious solution to man's problems seemed to be to use the same techniques on human beings as in cattle breeding.

'Positive' eugenics had a fairly brief history. Even if it is possible to agree on the desirability of different moral and intellectual traits,

* Lejeune – a distinguished French cytogeneticist – has argued that the nature of medicine is to work against natural selection in correcting genetical defects; when medicine is used to reinforce natural selection, it becomes eugenics and not medicine. The fallacy of this argument is that natural selection is a product of the physical and biological environment in which we live. Everything we do modifies this environment (see Hilton *et al.* 1973).

their genetic basis is almost completely unknown. Even worse, any genes concerned with such characteristics will be distributed throughout the genome, and could only be concentrated at the cost of unbalancing other developmental systems. Maynard Smith[9] has calculated that if one per cent of females with an IQ 100 had half their children by donors with an IQ 115, the mean of IQ of the population would rise by 0.04 points; if 10% of women opted for sperm from men of IQ 160, the rise would be 1.5 points. As Maynard Smith states that is 'almost certainly not worth the establishment of a new cult or religion'.

Negative eugenics has always seemed more feasible and a number of countries have eugenic sterilization laws on their statute books. However, these have a negligible effect even where they are enforced. Sterilization of carriers of dominantly-inherited conditions can reduce the incidence of the condition in question but cannot eliminate it, since many cases are due to new mutation. Sterilization of homozygotes for deleterious recessive genes would have a negligible effect on the large number of the genes present in the heterozygous state throughout the population (this is easily calculable from the Hardy-Weinberg equation). Even if heterozygotes could be detected, the fact that we all carry on average four or five deleterious recessive genes means that a concerted attack on all these at once would be somewhat drastic! Moreover, we know from the example of the sickle cell gene that many apparently pathogenic genes are not unconditionally harmful.

The Modern Phase

1. Modern interest in genetic engineering began with the idea of regulated *artificial insemination* borrowed from stock breeders. Specially selected donors might be used for artificial insemination for couples not satisfied with their own characteristics. The number of artificial inseminations already being carried out is unknown but there are at least 10,000 per year in the USA. If present attitudes to childlessness persists, the procedure will become more common and some sort of control of at least the source and storage of sperm will have to be instituted, although it seems unlikely that this will go as far as the 'National Pedigree Board' advocated by H. J. Müller. Children born following AID are technically illegitimate, although probably most of them are registered with the mother's husband as the named father.

2. Advances in reproductive physiology allow the *transplantation* of a fertilized ovum into a woman who might be sterile, or who might undertake the chore of pregnancy for another. *In vitro* separation of X- and Y- bearing sperm is probably near, permitting choice of sex for a child. This would probably produce an excess of males to satisfy parental wishes.

3. *Algeny* (or chemical control of the genotype) is the fanciful level

which probably means genetic engineering to most people. The first fruits of the microbiological manipulations now possible are likely to be the insertion of either artificial or human genes into viruses in order to produce, on a manufacturing scale, therapeutically important molecules such as insulin or growth hormone. The next step of inserting genes into patients with identifiable metabolic blocks will probably be realized in the foreseeable future. This is most likely to be achieved by infecting a culture of the patient's own cells with a 'repaired gene', and then inoculating him with the changed cells.

As a result of concern among some microbiologists about the possible hazards of pathogenic microorganisms carrying human genes a temporary moratorium on research on these lines was agreed some years ago. It is now generally accepted that these anxieties were exaggerated and research is now proceeding under an agreed code of practice.[10]

Other suggestions for algeny have been made, such as using repressor molecules to block the expression of certain characteristics or, even more radically, direct gene surgery on chromosomes by laser beams, etc. Essentially these techniques would lead to the early Mendelian hope of directed mutation. The problem always remains of damaging other genes than the one being 'operated on'.

Clonal Proliferation is, strictly speaking, a modification of the population phenotype rather than its genotype, (i.e. euthenics or euphenics, and not eugenics). It is comparable to vegetative reproduction which is widely used in horticulture to establish standard varieties. Since the nucleus of all cells in the body has an identical genetic complement, 'if a superior individual – and presumably genotype – is identified, why not copy it directly, rather than suffer all the risks, including those of sex determination, involved in the disruptions of recombination?'[11] In other words, take a body cell, and use it as a zygote by implanting it in the uterus. Since we can choose the individual from which the cell came:

a) There will be no risk of an inferior phenotype, which can only be recognized fifteen to twenty years after the original experiment.
b) There will be no problems with gene segregation or sex as in the normal recombinational lottery.
c) All the individuals produced will be genetically identical and hence have interchangeable parts.
d) There will be academic interest in comparing identical twins of different generations: will the second Einstein be better than the original?

Clonal proliferation is the theoretical goal of women's liberation, since it does away with the need for males; it has been described as auto-adultery. Indeed, it is the realization of the process described by Aldous Huxley in *Brave New World* where appropriate genotypes were bred for each job – epsilon demimorons for lift operators, and so on. The difficulty is that it completely avoids the question of the cumulative worth of a particular genotype over a lifetime.

Some of the Ethical Issues

It used to be thought that the genetic constitution of man was sacrosanct and could not be altered. With the discovery of chemically induced mutations and the metabolic reactions in gene-directed synthesis those ideas have had to be scrapped. Nevertheless, grandiose claims that we can now direct the future course of our evolution are facile. On the other hand, we may be unwise to regard the management of genetic disease as a problem no more difficult technically that that of managing – say – viral disease. The main difference between a bad gene and a bad germ is that one is an integral part of the human constitution whereas the other invades from outside. At the moment we have some prospect of eliminating an infection but we can only occasionally correct the damage done in an individual by genetic disorder. At present, our powers are mainly limited to recognizing it early and preventing the birth of the child concerned or palliating the effects in the living person.

Genetic disease may cause suffering through the physical and mental limitations it imposes on a patient, and it may shorten life. There are also burdens – sometimes heavy – which it places on others. Although suffering is inescapable in human life it can often be avoided or diminished. It is the accepted aim of the medical profession to reduce suffering without denying that it may have a creative value for those affected by it. It is one of the paradoxes of human existence that suffering refines character so that out of weakness comes unexpected strength. In other words, the physical difficulties of living and the personal experience of life need to be kept in balance; they are not necessarily equated.

We have in this chapter discussed some of the genetic problems which a doctor faces. His aim is clear and has been well summarized in the following words 'wherever and whenever possible our knowledge should be used to provide all children with the capacity for life without severe mental or physical defects and a measure of nurture and education that will enable them to achieve a full development of their capacities'.[12] As he sets about his task of reducing the effects of inherited disorders in both children and families he has to consider the methods at his disposal which are currently in use or likely to be developed (see section on 'genetic engineering'). He also has to consider the modification of gene-pools in different populations by voluntary or legalized eugenic programmes and by such factors as reduction in family size.

But medical decision must be subservient to our understanding of the nature of man himself. This will include the uniqueness and inestimable value of each individual life, the obligations of society to the individual and of the individual to society (a difficult balance to establish) and the use of education, persuasion and coercion (either legislative or social) to help individuals to make decisions in respect of genetic problems.

At the moment the most pressing problems concern abortions. The decision to ask for an abortion belongs to the parents and they will be influenced by their medical advisers whose attitude will be formed by social and religious factors as well as medical. As mentioned above (p. 42) the wish to have an infant physically whole need not override the desire to accept the new life as a divine gift even though deformity may be present. To many respect for human life is paramount.

If there is a probability of bearing a deformed child the parents may prefer to opt for childlessness or to plan for adoption, neither of which raise any immediate ethical issues. AID needs to be considered critically because the implications for society are far-reaching. Though not legally constituting adultery, children born as a result of it are technically illegitimate and, more significantly, may be regarded as a permanent intrusion into an established married relationship on a personal level. The fact that the identity of the donor is kept secret means that the child can never know who his father is. What is happening is a threat to the kinship structure of society and implies that biological fatherhood within marriage is something which can be safely discarded. Since the number of such births is increasing the effects on society will be cumulative. The other side of the picture must not be overlooked. Is it not a morally questionable act which allows a man to make a woman pregnant whom he can never know and become father to a child he will never see? This whole area of AID introduces a situation in which biological fatherhood and its attendant responsibilities can be deliberately thrown aside and needs to be treated with great caution. The many legal complications resulting from AID have yet to be resolved.

There are other far-reaching problems about the ethics of interference in reproductive and development processes, for every attempt to alter the pattern of family relationships sooner or later brings its backlash upon us. Is there a point at which we should say no? Ramsey,[13] for example, places the bar at what he calls the 'dehumanization of man'. This is fine in theory but leads to arbitrary rules in practice for who can say when a man is or is not human. Who can determine the limits of what is human life?

Robert Morison[14] (cited by Taylor 1968) writes 'once sex and reproduction are separated, society will have to struggle with defining the nature of interpersonal relationships which have no long-term social point . . . and seek new ways to ensure reasonable care for infants and children in an emotional atmosphere which lacks biological reinforcement'.

Surely, the doctor, above all others, is the guardian of life both in its biological uniqueness and in its natural human relationships? This concept has been at the heart of medical ethics in Western Civilization and must be preserved.

Glossary

AID: artificial insemination by donor.

Alleles: alternative version of a gene found at the same locus.

Amniocentesis: puncture of the amniotic sac to sample the fluid.

Aneuploid: where there are chromosome(s) additional to, or missing from, the normal diploid number of 46 in man.

Clone: all the cells derived from a single cell and carrying therefore identical genetic information.

Expressivity: the variability in effect of the same gene between individuals.

Gene: that section of the DNA molecule carrying information necessary for the synthesis of a specific polypeptide.

Genetic load: the total of harmful genes affecting either individuals or particular populations.

Genome: the whole genetic information of an individual.

Genotype: the genetic constitution of an individual at a particular locus.

Heterozygote (heterozygous): where there are different alleles at the same locus of a corresponding/homologous pair of chromosomes.

Homozygote (homozygous): where there is the same allele at the corresponding locus of a pair of chromosomes.

Locus: position of a gene on a chromosome.

Multifactorial: where many factors, both genetic and environmental, usually each of small effect, are involved.

Mutation (point mutation): change in a single gene.

Phenotype: the actual appearance of an individual.

Reduced penetrance: when not all individuals carrying a gene show clinical evidence of it.

Translocated chromosome: where part of one chromosome has become transferred to another.

Zygote: the fertilized egg.

References

1. Sorenson, J. R. (1971) *Social Aspects of Applied Human Genetics*. New York, Sage.
2. Carter, C. O., Roberts, J. A. F., Evans, K. A. & Buck, A. R. (1971) Genetic counselling: a follow-up. *Lancet*, 1, 281–5.
3. Lubs, H. A. (1973) Privacy and genetic information. In Hilton, *et al.*, pp. 267–75.

4. Mikelsaar, A. V. N. *et al.* (1975) Human karyotype polymorphism. *Humangenetik*, **26**, 1–23, these workers showed that minor chromosomal variants are found more frequently in mentally retarded than in normal people.
5. Gendel, E., Weingold, A. B., Elaquin, F. & Kim, H. S. (1972) E trisomy diagnosed *in utero*. *New England Journal of Medicine* **287**, 995–6.
6. Scriver, C. R. (1972) Screening for inherited traits: perspectives. In *Early Diagnosis of Human Genetics Traits* (Harris, M. (Ed.)), pp. 87–98. Bethesda, Maryland, National Institutes of Health.
7. Borgaonkar, B. S. & Shah, S. A. (1974) The XYY chromosome male – or syndrome. *Progress in Medical Genetics* **10**, 135–222.
8. e.g. Penrose, L. S. (1955) Evidence of heterosis in man. *Proceedings of the Royal Society, B*, **144**, 203–213.
9. Smith, J. M. (1965) Eugenics and Utopia. *Daedalus*, **94**, 487–505.
10. Ashby Report (1975) *Report of the Working Party on the Experimental Manipulation of the Genetic Composition of Microorganisms*. Cmnd 5880. London, HMSO.
11. Lederberg, J. (1966) Experimental genetics and human evolution. *American Naturalist*, **100**, 519–531.
12. World Council of Churches (1974) *Genetics and the Quality of Life*. Geneva, W.C.C.
13. Ramsey, P. (1970) *Fabricated Man. The Ethics of Genetic Control*. New Haven & London, Yale University Press.
14. Taylor, G. R. (1968) *The Biological Time Bomb*. London, Thames and Hudson, p. 179.

Further Reading

Anderson, J. N. D. (1976) *Issues of Life and Death*. London, Hodder and Stoughton.

Baer, A. S., (Ed.) (1973) *Heredity and Society. Readings in Social Genetics*. New York, Macmillan.

Birch, C. & Abrecht, P., (Eds.) (1975) *Genetics and the Quality of Life*. Oxford, Pergamon.

Fletcher, J. (1974) *The Ethics of Genetic Control*. New York, Doubleday.

Harris, H. (1974) *Prenatal Diagnosis and Selective Abortion*. London, Nuffield Provincial Hospitals Trust.

Hilton, B., Callahan, D., Harris, M., Condliffe, P. & Berkley, B. (Eds.) (1973) *Ethical Issues in Human Genetics*. New York, Plenum.

Jones, A. & Bodmer, W. F. (1974) *Our Future Inheritance: Choice or Chance?* London, Oxford University Press.

Ramsey, P. (1970) *Fabricated Man. The Ethics of Genetic Control*. New York and London, Yale University Press.

Veatch, R. M. (1974) Ethical issues in genetics. *Progress in Medical Genetics*. **10**, 223–264.

5

The Control of the Beginning of Life

Introduction
Gordon Scorer and Antony Wing

No subjects have been more freely discussed during the past two or three decades than contraception and abortion. They lie at the heart of medical ethics for they concern man and woman at the point where life begins. It is here that biological pressures and emotional sensibilities are so extraordinarily powerful. Yet instinct must be guided and we are all free to act as we choose. Who controls public opinion – and by what right? Its influence on young minds in matters of sex may be decisive for good or evil. What ought the doctor to be thinking about these matters? He is frequently asked to advise or prescribe.

But neither contraception nor abortion can be considered in isolation. Both are closely related to the way men, women and children live together in families and both are strongly influenced by what has recently come to be regarded as a topic in its own right – 'sex education'. Our understanding of family life, contraception and abortion is conditioned by the kind of education we receive. And here it is not biological facts that matter so much as attitude to life in its essential nature and in its personal relationships.

The Present Position   It is difficult to exaggerate the effect of the sexual revolution which swept over the Western World in the 1960s. Stemming in part from Freud's view that many adult neuroses arise from sexual experiences in childhood, the movement towards 'sexual freedom' was powerfully boosted by Kinsey's publications on sexual behaviour in males and females. Two large volumes appeared in America purporting to give details of normal intimate sexual activity unseen by the public eye. Almost overnight sex-conduct became a world-wide talking point.

With the discovery and marketing of the contraceptive pill as almost one hundred per cent effective and allegedly causing negligible side effects, the world was offered the possibility – for the first time in history – of fully separating sexual intercourse from the conception of new life (procreation). Propoganda was intensive. Very soon sex activity was presented as an end in itself, as a 'good' to be sought for its own sake, as a necessary step towards maturity in the adolescent and as an essential part of healthy living in the adult. It was no wonder young people were bemused.

In the meanwhile it had become apparent that the number of illegal abortions being carried out in the country was increasing.

54

More babies were being conceived within and outside marriage which were 'not wanted'. The Abortion Act of 1967, the result of a well-planned campaign over the previous 30 years, extended the grounds on which a pregnancy could be legally terminated. From then on the number of legal abortions rose rapidly and eventually levelled off in 1974 at over 100,000 a year. Despite the popularization of the contraceptive pill and the fact that it can be obtained free of charge, the number of abortions has not declined appreciably. It is considered that abortion must remain 'an essential back-stop' to help those who have failed in their contraceptive precautions or do not wish to use them.

Interlinked with these facts about contraception and abortion is the rapid rise in the past few years in the divorce rate (now running at 125,000 a year with almost one in two marriages breaking down in those who marry under 25). Family life is disintegrating, single parent families are increasing and the responsibilities of fatherhood are being abdicated. Into this situation the doctor is drawn – often as an unwilling participant. He is sympathetic to human need but singularly helpless against the disruptive forces currently over-whelming society. What ought he to think? How ought he to act when the patient comes to him expecting something to be done which he, as a doctor, alone can do?

Family limitation may be achieved by self control. Until recently this has probably been the commonest method used. Since, however, it is so often either unacceptable or a failure, both abortion and infanticide have been practised throughout human history with varying degrees of public tolerance. It is only in the past century that increasingly sophisticated contraceptive techniques have been introduced and, because their succesful use involves a knowledge of human anatomy and physiology, the doctor's role has become of paramount importance. Abortion and sterilization being now legal under certain conditions they too, must be medically controlled. The doctor therefore finds himself confronted by ethical problems which he does not find easy to resolve.

It will always be the first duty of the doctor to protect human life especially when it is most vulnerable. And yet this cannot be effec-tively done unless the human relationships which surround its procreation and nurture are strong and enduring. Education for sex is a damaging concept if it becomes isolated as a subject in its own right. It is essential, therefore, that children are brought up to respect one another and to value the realities of marriage and family life in which alone the physical and emotional aspects of biological sex can safely mature.

59722

Contraception and Sterilization
Hugh Handley Bird and William Sinclair

Methods of contraception, their side effects, complications and failure rate are not considered here as such information can be obtained from many freely available publications. Suffice it to say that fertility varies enormously between married couples. There are some who are burdened with high fertility – 'Can you help me doctor? I have only got to shake hands with my wife and she gets pregnant'. Others are cursed with infertility – 'I would give anything in the world to have children'.

Contraception within Marriage

Religious and ethical views are here closely interlinked and may be considered together. Contraception is not an issue discussed in the Bible. Children are regarded as a gift of God – especially in the Old Testament – a sign of His blessing on the tribe and on the individual. When God at Creation blessed man and woman and said to them 'be fruitful and multiply and fill the earth and subdue it and have dominion . . .'[1] the words appear to have been spoken more as a promise to be realized and a prospect to be enjoyed than a command to be blindly carried out. In the power he gave man, God offered a blessing not a curse. It is no part of the divine mandate that the earth should be over-populated or its natural resources destroyed.

The incident recorded in Genesis,[2] of the divine judgment on Onan is because of an act of coitus interruptus. It has usually been interpreted as a condemnation of the practice. The context, however, is important and gives a clue to the cause of the divine anger. God's judgment was not because Onan used this particular contraceptive method but because he failed to fulfil the law of Moses which was designed to ensure that his sister-in-law would have children and thus continue his dead brother's family line.

The Roman Catholic Church officially permits only the use of the rhythm method as a means of avoiding pregnancy. Pope Paul VI in his encyclical letter of 1968[3] reiterated the Vatican's opposition to all other methods. This has created wide-spread opposition within the Roman Catholic community from both laity and clergy. As far back as 1930[4] the Lambeth Conference of Anglican Bishops reversed its previous attitude of disapproval of the use of artificial contraceptive methods. Certainly most religious bodies would consider it responsible rather than sinful for a husband and wife to plan the procreative aspect of sexual relationship, while continuing to enjoy the physical or 'unitive' side of marriage.

Married partners are often influenced in their choice of family planning technique by the way in which it operates. For example, many will find acceptable a method which prevents fertilization occurring, but will reject one which allows fertilization to take place and then destroys the fertilized ovum.[5] Some – particularly Christians – may avoid the pill just because it interferes fundamentally with normal menstrual physiology and carries its own risks to health. The point at issue is that many within the churches (especially Roman Catholic, Eastern or Orthodox) cannot accept that man has a right to modify or artificially control *the essential physiological activity of human procreation.*

It appears, however, that the use of contraceptives within marriage is, in general, accepted by Christians as a means of enhancing their married unity but not for selfish ends. If, therefore, contraceptive practice fails (as sometimes it will) the result is an unexpected pregnancy but is not an *unwanted* child. Rather, the new life is gladly accepted.

Usually, no doctor will experience any special difficulty in discussing freely with his married patient the methods and problems of contraceptive use. The acceptability of his advice is bound to depend upon the degree of Christian understanding and commitment of the one he is talking to.

Contraception outside marriage

It is here that the major ethical problems arise. They often present the doctor with an acute dilemma – to prescribe or not to prescribe. The law of the land does not compel a doctor to become involved in work of this nature, but it is usually difficult for him to opt out of it, and he may not wish to do so.

Where the patient is under the age of consent the problem increases. Sexual intercourse under sixteen years of age is illegal and therefore the law may become involved. Moreover, there is the additional difficulty relating to parental permission; most parents would wish to know what their young daughters are doing in this respect. Early teenage pregnancy is a disaster, probably leaving life-long physical and psychological damage. What shall the doctor's attitude be?

Social Pressures Today

Social influences – that is, what the majority of people consider is the right way to behave – in most matters work strongly in a doctor's favour. The sick come to him for advice, comfort and practical help, because men and women everywhere want to be well. The public are on the side to the doctor in his intentions to relieve or to cure. On the other hand the modern sexual revolution, is so far as it has captured and is controlling public opinion, is having a disruptive effect on society. Too often it tries to compel the doctor to support attitudes and practices which he knows to be against the best interests of young people, family life and the welfare of children.

The story of the Family Planning Association offers the best illustration of what is happening today. Starting in 1930 as the National Birth Control Council its purpose was to spread the knowledge of birth control methods and to educate women in how to limit the size of their family by the use of contraceptives. Just before the last war the Council changed its name to Family Planning Association but its function remained the same. It was concerned to advise and help those who were married or were about to be married.

Once the climate of opinion began to alter, the Association accommodated itself to the new views. It became caught up in the propaganda machine which defended the right of *young unmarried people* to become sexually experienced on the ground that, provided a pregnancy did not occur and provided they did not damage one another, no harm would occur. By implication sexual activity from early teens onward became accepted as both natural and inevitable, irrespective of the personal commitment and bond of marriage. The propaganda became a vicious spiral. The more young people were encouraged to become sexually active the more necessary it was to educate them in the use of contraceptives to prevent pregnancy. Yet the more these matters were brought to their notice at 'educational level' the more they became interested, aroused and then eager participators. Since young people naturally found their parents opposed to this damaging exploitation of physical relationships the propaganda was turned against parents who were represented as out of date, oppressive or dangerous in their views. The glossy magazines, in a constant stream of attractive articles read by vast numbers of children and teenagers, offer advice based on the importance of sexual adventure as a natural and glamorous thing to do.[6]

The number of women using contraceptives has, of course, risen enormously, but the fact that the pill can be obtained free of charge (unlike ordinary medical prescriptions) implies that sexual activity outside marriage meets with Government approval and must therefore be regarded as 'normal'. The widespread use of the pill among teenagers and schoolgirls is common knowledge. It is no wonder that the pregnancy rate in unmarried girls has risen – particularly in the 16 to 19 age group – and that the abortion rate among those in their *early* teens has also reached an alarming level.

In 1971 an investigation[7] was carried out in Aberdeen University into the sexual behaviour and contraceptive practice of unmarried female undergraduates. 90% of the sample replied and of these 44% had experienced sexual intercourse in the previous six weeks. The authors pleaded for easier access to contraceptive advice and supplies and deplored any doctor's hesitation in acceding to a girl's request.

A courageous commentary appeared a few weeks later in the same journal[8] written by a woman doctor who was an adviser to the students. 'Young women at the universities nowadays,' she wrote, 'are at the mercy of a virulent environment. They are daily – and at all hours – in the company of eager young men. . . . The women are thrown into situations of unpremeditated sexual arousal'. Although she said she was willing to give contraceptive advice, every request gave her a pang because it was 'just another condonation of a social development which, by all the standards I know and by all the wisdom I can summon seems erroneous – for individuals and for the ultimate good of the community'.

Most doctors are daily reminded of the break-up of family life in the nation today consequent upon the loss of the old moral standards which used to bind people together in mutual respect and with a will to safeguard the issues of life and death. The individual practitioner may indeed be forgiven if he feels isolated and oppressed standing alone against an apparently irresistible tide.

Possible Solutions

It is generally agreed that when a girl asks for a prescription for the contraceptive pill she has either had sexual experience or intends to get it. Her mind is usually made up – but not always.

Those doctors who take a broadly permissive attitude and often help when asked, have to answer the fact that – moral, spiritual and social considerations apart – the pill is not without its damaging effects in the physically immature. In addition, psychological problems, sexual inadequacy and frustration have greatly increased among the unmarried. Very many who experiment when young find it difficult to make lasting and meaningful relations when they do wish to settle in marriage.

It is not possible either logically or practically for the doctor to maintain a neutral position – saying it is the girl's decision not his. A patient comes to the doctor knowing that he has the authority and experience to prescribe effective drugs and has the competence to do so. The giving of a prescription implies that the doctor supports the use to which the drug is going to be put. Even a shopkeeper may not sell to a client what he knows will be harmful.

Reluctant agreement to prescribe on the grounds that the girl will get the pills anyway, or if she does not there may be an unwanted pregnancy, sounds plausible but it underestimates the doctor's moral influence and authority with his patients. Many a girl has been grateful for a doctor's sympathy and his realistic presentation of the other side.

The situationist argument – that where true love is there no rules should be allowed – flies in the face of all human experience. True love knows how to wait. Love in the absence of moral standards and disciplined living can be destructive; it is not absolute. Moreover the argument overlooks the human tendency to rationalize evil acts and persuade himself that they are good.

The Christian Position   The Christian position is that sexual intercourse is reserved for marriage. There alone it finds its true meaning both in the fulfilment of individual personality and in the strengthening of the love bond. Moreover, the social benefits of such enduring relationships are incalculable. In any interview, if the girl admits to being a Christian, discussion can progress in a positive direction. Christianity is not a rigid moral code which is both theoretical and impracticable, rather it offers spiritual insight and resources beyond the normal capacity of men and women.

General Attitudes   On the other hand, for those who oppose these truths and do not believe that God has any place in the contract of marriage (and may even deny that the State has any right in it either) the problem may be seen otherwise. There are some doctors who, knowing that the relationship is intended to be permanent – and therefore complies with an elementary notion of what marriage is all about – are prepared to prescribe on that assumption. To those who contemplate no permanent relationship the harm of what they are doing to themselves and their partner needs to be mentioned. A doctor is not compelled to prescribe against his better judgment.

None dare estimate the magnitude of the social changes which have so remarkably captured the minds of young people in the name of freedom and progress. Nevertheless the situation is not irreversible. The doctor's concern to promote and encourage all that is best in family life is a powerful weapon in his hand. As a continuing, compassionate adviser of what he knows to be right he is a bulwark against sexual anarchy and its attendant miseries.

Sterilization

Sterilization is intended to be permanent contraception. In the female tubal ligation can be easily performed two or three days after childbirth or as an interval procedure unrelated to pregnancy. There may be sound arguments for postponing the operation for a few months for the reason that a woman's decision may be emotionally prejudiced immediately after the birth of her baby – or the baby may die in infancy.

The operation entails a general anaesthetic, an abdominal operation and a stay in hospital for a period varying from a few hours to a week, depending on the technique used. In the male vasectomy is a simpler method of sterilization not requiring a general anaesthetic, which can be performed, therefore, on an out-patient basis.

Both methods are almost completely reliable and are, of course, usually permanent. This finality is one argument against it, in that in the event of the death of the spouse, or divorce, the sterilized partner may re-marry and wish to have a child. Operations to reverse sterilization are difficult, and the success rate even in experienced hands, is at present poor.

Another disadvantage may be the emotional one. Most marriages improve after sterilization as the couple are able to enjoy intercourse without fear of pregnancy. In a minority of cases, however, the absence of risk removes the thrill of sexual relationship, the wife loses her libido and the marriage deteriorates.

A third argument sometimes raised against sterilization is an ethical one. It allows the sterilized man or woman freedom to have sexual relationships at any time with another partner without the possibility of pregnancy occurring. Gynaecologists are becoming familiar with the 'failed vasectomy – pregnant wife' syndrome. Usually the husband is found to be azoospermic, the pregnancy being the result of an extra-marital relationship.

Some oppose sterilization on religious grounds (because of the damage done to *normal* anatomy and physiology) and this is the official Roman Catholic view. A therapeutic sterilization may rightly be done when further child bearing could damage the mother's health or risk her life.

Sterilization of the Mentally Ill (see p. 132)

This may raise difficult ethical problems especially if the patient is mentally subnormal *and* a minor. The matter was highlighted in 1975 by the publicity surrounding an 11-year-old Sheffield girl whose operation was forbidden by a Court Order. The issue here is that children below the age of 16 are not, by law, considered old enough to give consent to an operation. In addition, the operation is not therapeutic but is done for personal and social reasons. Many gynaecologists will say it is wrong to operate in such cases in any circumstances; it is better to try to educate the child, or persuade her, if need be, to use contraceptives (possibly injectable ones) or to carry out an abortion.[9] Parental ability to persuade, even in the mentally subnormal, may be surprisingly effective.

On the other hand there are all degrees of mental subnormality, and Gardner[10] does not consider that it is always realistic to refuse sterilization, for there are cases where a severely retarded girl, even under close parental or institutional care, has become pregnant. It is important that any such operation undertaken on someone who is unable to give consent should be discussed on as broad a basis as possible with all those who have the welfare of the patient at heart. What is not legally permissible is for the doctor on his own clinical judgment to carry out a sterilization operation on a minor even with the parents consent.[11]

Indications for non-Therapeutic Sterilization

Sir Dugald Baird[12] in his Sandoz Foundation lecture 'The Fifth Freedom', suggested that it was time to give freedom from the tyranny of excessive fertility a place alongside the other well-known 'four freedoms', But the reverse is also true – the freedom to bear a child, especially at this juncture in our national life when advocates of birth-prevention have so much to say.

In the Aberdeen Maternity Hospital the criteria used by Baird when assessing a patient for tubal ligation were wise and balanced. At one time these criteria were: age at least 25 years, four children and a stable marriage, but opinions are bound to change constantly and gynaecologists will vary their indications for sterilization to suit circumstances. Many now advise performing a postpartum sterilization following the birth of a second child, but it must be remembered that healthy baby at birth is not a guarantee of survival as the first year of life is still a period of high risk.

Summary

The population explosion has intensified the discussion on family limitation and in some countries made it a matter of urgency. In the developed countries it can be argued that despite a static birth rate, each new child is going to use a disproportionate amount of the world's irreplaceable raw materials. In the developing countries where the population may have doubled in the last 25 years the problem is usually one of undernourishment and the possibility of starvation. These facts do not *dictate* family size but every couple will wish to take into account social and economic factors when they plan their family. The ethical question as to whether a couple have an indisputable right to decide their family size has yet to be openly debated.

References

1. Genesis 1, 28.
2. Genesis 38, 7–10.
3. Encyclical letter of Pope Paul VI *Humanae Vitae*, 1968.
4. Lambeth Conference 1930. Encyclical letter from the Bishops with resolution and reports. London, 1930.
5. A full discussion on this and allied subjects is given in Gardner, R. F. R. (1973) *Moral Dilemmas in Contraceptive Developments*. London, Christian Medical Fellowship.

6. Nash, Joanna (1975) *Entertainment or Exploitation. A critical survey of Girls' Teenage Magazines.* The Responsible Society.
7. McCance, C. & Hall, D. J. (1972) *British Medical Journal,* **2,** 694.
8. Anderson, Violet (1972) Personal View.*British Medical Journal,* **3,** 524.
9. *Journal of Medical Ethics.* (1975) Child Sterilization **1,** 163.
10. Gardner, R. F. R. (1976) *Journal of Medical Ethics,* **2,** 99.
11. For an excellent summary of the present situation, see Thomson, W. A. R. (1977) *Medical Ethics and Practice.* Bristol, John Wright.
12. Baird, Sir Dugald (1965) *British Medical Journal,* **2,** 1141.

The Termination of Pregnancy
Rex Gardner

Abortion is the loss of the embryo or fetus from the womb of the mother, before it can live independently – that is, before about the 22nd week of gestation. If such an occurrence is unintended it is defined as an 'accidental' or 'spontaneous' abortion or, in lay terms, a 'miscarriage'. This latter term is to be preferred because it causes no offence to the disappointed parents and it is unambiguous.

If the abortion is procured by an act of interference to the womb it is an 'induced' abortion or more simply, a termination of the pregnancy. In this instance it may be 'therapeutic' if done to save the life or health of the mother, 'legal' when the act falls within the terms of current legislation on the matter, or 'illegal' or 'criminal' if it falls outside them.

Abortion, the deliberate termination of a pregnancy, has been practised from time immemorial. It was either done by the mother herself or by an accomplice. The usual motive being either to hide a clandestine sexual relationship, or to prevent an additional burden to an already overstretched family. In recent decades the law against medically induced abortion has been relaxed in most countries of the world. It is widely practised to prevent the birth of a child likely to be disadvantaged by one of the following conditions: congenital malformation, mental inadequacy, the stigma of illegitimacy, or, simply because it is unwanted. It has also been advocated as a backstop to failed contraception, or even as an essential and permanent partner, with contraception, in any serious attempt to halt the population explosion.[1] Many today consider that every woman should have the right to a termination of her pregnancy if she wishes – but the ethical problems arising from such an attitude are many and far-reaching.

The 1967 Act

In Britain, without legal sanction but in reliance on the acquittal of a gynaecologist who aborted a raped minor,[2] terminations of pregnancy for severe maternal ill-health were being openly performed in NHS hospitals for many years, before 1967. At the same time, with the support of co-operative psychiatrists, a few liberal-minded operators were performing terminations on less well-defined grounds in the private sector. A satisfactory legal framework for the operation was therefore advocated in order to get rid of what was becoming 'one law for the rich and another for the poor'. Also, it was needed in order that the rising number of dangerous, sometimes fatal, back-street abortions could be replaced by safe, free operations performed by competent gynaecologists. In these circumstances the Abortion Act of 1967 was passed by the parliament of the United Kingdom.

Under this Act abortion is not illegal if, before it is undertaken, two registered medical practitioners (neither of whom need be the actual operator) have certified in good faith (a) that the continuance of the pregnancy would involve risk to the life of the pregnant woman, or of injury to the physical or mental health of the pregnant woman, or of any existing children of the family, greater than if the pregnancy were terminated or (b) that there is a substantial risk that if the child were born it would suffer from such physical or mental abnormalities as to be seriously handicapped. It is further laid down that, in reaching a decision, account may be taken of the pregnant woman's actual or reasonably foreseeable environment.

Ethical Issues

Ethical attitudes to abortion turn on the relative weight in argument given to the fetus, to the mother, to society and the moral law.

Fetus-centered Views

Where the fetus is considered to be *a human life*, or even a person in the full sense of the word[3] abortion may be seen as 'murder'. This viewpoint, however, would appear untenable as it is of the essence of murder that there must be malice toward the victim. If it is the *well-being of the mother* which is the prime consideration, the intention cannot be counted as evil.

Some consider the fetus to be inviolable under all circumstances. Others, including most Roman Catholic moralists, consider it to be inviolable to direct assault, but justifiably sacrificed if this is an unavoidable consequence of the surgical extirpation of some potentially fatal condition of the genital tract, for example uterine cancer, or a diseased fallopian tube containing ectopic gestation.[4] Many authorities widen this viewpoint to allow direct attack on the fetus if continuation of the pregnancy would gravely endanger the mother's life. Judge Macnaughten in the Bourne case however, held that termination of the pregnancy to prevent the girl becoming a mental wreck could be construed as saving her life.[5]

Once abortion is permitted to save the health as well as the life of the mother, the insoluble problem arises of defining 'health'. It is impossible to distinguish ill-health due to demonstrable physical pathology from that due to a mental disorder. It is found in experience that there is a continuous spectrum starting with such a clear-cut case as the woman who would, by continued pregnancy, suffer a most serious physical deterioration (such as renal failure), and ending with the woman who would suffer a transitory mild depression. Nowhere on the spectrum is a clear cut-off point to be found.

Mother-centred Views

Many brush aside all argument, holding that the mother has an absolute right over her own body. They see the fetus as a mass of cells within that body, disposable at the mother's discretion, if unwanted, in the same way as is her appendix. This viewpoint is unacceptable chiefly because it ignores the fact that the fetus does not consist of maternal cells but has its own genetic constitution and because from the beginning of the second trimester it is fully formed requiring only maternal nutrition and protection. It also begs the question of when the fetus is truly unwanted. Pregnant women suffer considerable fluctuations in mood, largely in response to swiftly changing hormonal levels, as a result of which their attitude to their pregnancy varies from day to day. It has been maintained that the unwanted child has an increased risk of non-accidental injury. The study of baby-battering parents does not bear this out.[6] Others suggest that abortion is itself the ultimate in baby-battering!

A polarization of attitudes easily occurs. On the one hand the advocates of easily available abortion usually start from the woman's view-point and pay no attention to the fetus. Their opponents feel that such a cavalier attitude to another life – albeit only potential – will readily lead to an attitude which regards the unwanted, the weak, the unfit and the inconvenient members of society as disposable. Such a cheapening of human life could, they say, bear ominous threat to the respect which society should always hold for human life.[7]

On the other hand, those who refuse to sanction abortion focus their attention on the fetus and pay scant regard to the mother and her existing family. They may carry this to an extreme point and deny life to a gravely ill mother. In such a case the fetus almost invariably succumbs so no life is in fact being saved by this attitude: the mother being sacrificed to save the conscience of a third party. In less severe cases the existing children of the woman may be so much disadvantaged by the illness of mother or the arrival of a further sibling, that they become deprived. They may start on the vicious circle[8] which leads through disturbed teenage to the inadequate adult, who in turn becomes an unsatisfactory parent generating unwanted pregnancies.

The Social Realities

The necessary consideration of the socio-economic conditions complicate decision making. The poverty-stricken woman working long hours to earn enough money to keep her family above the breadline, becomes worn out with backache from her toil and anaemic from her poor diet. The single girl may become chronically depressed from failure. In an attempt to prove herself lovable she becomes involved in a series of liaisons which so often end in desertion that she contemplates suicide from a sense of emptiness and despair – of which the pregnancy is merely a symptom, not the cause.

Such conditions make it difficult for the gynaecologist to take a 'tough-minded' yes or no decision on 'tender-minded' data, that is when there are no clear-cut or agreed norms.[9] In these circumstances a wide variation in practice has developed.

On the one hand there are those who terminate the pregnancies of relatively few women, interpreting the legal criteria strictly. They are criticized because those whom they refuse to help may become involved in the expenses of finding a private abortion at a distance or, worse, may in desperation be driven into the incompetent and potentially fatal hands of a back-street operator.

On the other hand there are others who practise abortion 'on demand', and who justify their practice by the fallacious statistical argument that as the abortion of any early pregnancy is less risky than that of normal delivery, every abortion falls within the meaning of the Act. They can be criticized for jeopardizing the girl's future obstetric performance due to post-infective infertility, or by the creation of cervical incompetence leading to second trimester miscarriage, or by rhesus sensitization. They are also accused of trivializing pregnancy and intercourse with potentially dire effects on the stability of the girl's marriage, and with an inevitable lowering of the moral standards of the nation.

Many doctors who do not like 'abortion on request' nevertheless feel that they are in no position to assess the many non-medical factors involved in the woman's predicament and abdicate responsibility, leaving the decision regarding abortion to the patient. One has known patients, however, who have afterwards volunteered that they were mentally bemused and had been in no fit state to come to such a decision. Especially is this so when they are under severe pressure from husband, boy-friend, or mother to have the operation. The help of trained counsellors is invaluable here in helping the woman to an understanding of her situation and of the fact that there is more than one option open. Such counselling is costly of time and effort. It must make available alternative accommodation if the girl is disowned at home, and on-going support is needed whatever action may be taken.

Gestational age is of great importance, and even doctors who are prepared to abort on request usually place an upper limit, often twelve weeks. Ethical and medical difficulties increase as the fetus gets older and larger. To act early in pregnancy is medically safer and may be ethically more acceptable.

Moral Standards in Society

What is socially acceptable – that is to say 'what is normally done in these circumstances' – has a powerful influence on personal decisions when a moral dilemma arises. The Abortion Act of 1967 has probably had the effect of making the termination of pregnancy acceptable to a majority in modern society. Law does not merely reflect public opinion, it moulds and redirects it. But the Act only permitted termination in certain circumstances; it is still illegal to destroy unborn life.

Uneasiness over the Act is likely to continue. Of course it may be argued that abortions have always occurred in every society and that it is only right that, if they are done, they should be made as safe as possible. But at a time when simple, effective and widely acceptable contraceptives are available why should the abortion figures continue to be so alarmingly high?

There appears to be at least three reasons. The current decline in moral standards means that there is little restraint in extra-marital sexual experiment. For this many girls are unprepared because of ignorance, or the unexpectedness of the occasion, or because the emotional cost of contraception in destroying their self-image is too great. Those with the knowledge and equipment for contraception frequently do not employ it because the back-stop of abortion makes the risk appear worth taking. The existence of contraception has so altered marriage as to make an unplanned pregnancy intolerable. When therefore there is a contraceptive 'slip-up' this unplanned pregnancy is no longer acceptable and abortion is sought.

The distinction between contraception and abortion, much emphasized by pioneers in contraception, has been denied by recent protagonists. Certainly the decision has been blurred by hind-sight contraception such as stilbestrol and the much publicized menstrual-evacuation techniques in which the uterus is emptied after the end of the cycle – no questions being asked as to its contents. Views on the morality of such techniques must depend on the significance placed on the early embryo.[10] The danger is always of the trivialization of human relationships, a reduction in respect for human life and the loosening of family-bonding to the impoverishment of man, woman and their children.

In Romania and other countries in Eastern Europe permissive abortion legislation has had to be repealed owing to an alarming fall in the birthrate.

The Influence of Religious Belief

Special difficulties arise for those who face the problem from a religious background. To the Christian conscience unavoidable destruction of life – even of unborn life at the earliest stages – can never become acceptable. To many Christians the only exceptions are where the mother's life or health are threatened or the infant is likely to be born with serious handicap. The planning of pregnancy is part and parcel of adult human responsibility in the marriage relationships. Population pressures and limited personal resources demand limitation of family size and we now have sophisticated means to achieve this for all who need them. Sexual intercourse outside marriage is not a Christian option whatever public opinion may suggest through the media.

Nevertheless, Christian doctors have to come to terms with the fact that they live in a real world. Some may consider it their duty not to be in any way involved with pregnancy termination except perhaps for the clearest medical indications. The desperate plight of girls who have become victims of a selfish and permissive age, the immature, the rejected, the inadequate and the unsupported most surely need compassionate help. And that help includes education, patient understanding, wise counselling and often financial support – as well as a doctor's actions on her behalf. For some this may involve arranging or performing a termination of pregnancy. Each involved doctor has to work out for himself what principles will guide him to make his decisions – but the long-term interests of the mother, the baby, the family and society need to be taken into consideration in forming his policy. In so doing he will be putting the patient's interests first and demonstrating his total concern for her good.

Hard Cases

The young, unmarried pregnant teenager presents a particularly difficult problem. Pregnancy and delivery may be hazardous, but termination may be even more so, being technically difficult, potentially jeopardizing future fertility and often emotionally traumatic. If she goes on with the pregnancy, her mother will in all probability have to bring up the child. However, such girls have, in our experience, a great inborn reluctance to abortion and often fight to continue their pregnancy against strong parental opposition.

Arguments concerning mental sequelae are double-edged. We have known women depressed when abortion has been refused and others depressed because it has been performed. Statistics for and against have been produced and reviewed. They prove to be of little value, however, as they deal with the problem only in psychiatric terms, no account being taken of the deeper and more important matter of the burdened conscience. Any discussion which leaves this factor out of account is incomplete and its claim to be scientific must be rebuffed. The suggestion that a sense of guilt is merely iatrogenic is completely unfounded. The effect of abortion on marital stability has to be judged in each case individually. In our experience there have been terminations which have saved marriages, and others which have destroyed them.

The Conscience Clause

A further problem is that legal safeguards built into the 1967 Act for members of the medical profession with conscientious objections against involvement in abortion have proved inadequate. Promotion to senior grades in gynaecology and anaesthesia has, as a result, proved very difficult, if not impossible for them.

Nurses often find it difficult to opt out of the care of these patients. It may be particularly repugnant to them and can be emotionally devastating for the woman herself, if a fetus, showing signs of life, is born in the ward following the use of prostaglandins to interrupt a second trimester pregnancy. For this reason, as well as the increased possibility of the now fully-formed child living, many operators rarely terminate a pregnancy beyond its twelfth week. Prior to this a relatively simple suction evacuation is usually possible.

Fetal Abnormalities

It had been hoped that one result of the Act would be a great diminution in the number of children born with congenital abnormalities. This has not proved to be the case, largely because few of them can be identified prior to birth. Mothers who suffer from rubella early in pregnancy are usually offered termination if they have a rising titre of rubella antibodies. Women in whom there is a known possibility of a genetic anomaly, and those over thirty-five whose risk of bearing a mongol child is high, are usually offered amniocentesis around the 16th week of pregnancy (see pp. 42–85). Women in whom a raised serum alphafetoprotein level suggests that the fetus has a major neural tube defect, such as spina bifida or anencephaly, come in this category. The procedure carries some risk and should not be undertaken unless the woman, knowing that the result indicated an affected child, would wish for a termination. The argument here is that it would be better for the child's sake not to be born, than to be born deformed. Some moralists have poured scorn on the idea.[11] It has been pointed out, moreover, that many normal fetuses are being aborted on the mere presumption of abnormality and some have been miscarried due to the trauma of the investigation. Because cell culture takes time it may not be possible to abort the affected fetus around the twentieth week.

In pregnancy termination for fetal abnormality there is a wide spectrum of ethical opinion to be considered as well as the nature of the congenital disorder to be discussed. At one extreme is the anencephalic which is incapable of existence and at the other is the fetus who happens to be of the sex which the parents do not wish to have. The problems of the mongol, the child with spina bifida and of aborting for the sex-linked diseases are such that there is unlikely to be unanimity of opinion among parents and doctors. For those in the Christian tradition the religious understanding of the value of unborn life will always lead them to be very reluctant to interfere except on firm diagnosis of a serious condition and after all discussion with paediatrician and the parents.

To date, all attempts to amend the Abortion Act of 1967 in order to provide better defined criteria for the termination of pregnancy have failed. Once any such an act is on the Statute Book it seems unlikely that its wording, however carefully framed, can hold the floodgates against those determined to abort at will.

References

1. Potts, M., Diggory, P. & Peel, J. (1977) *Abortion*: Cambridge University Press.
2. Bourne, A. (1963) *A Doctor's Creed: The Memoirs of a Gynaecologist*. London, Gollancz.
3. Bajema, C. E. (1974) *Abortion and the Meaning of Personhood*. Grand Rapids; Baker Book House.
4. Haring, B. (1972) *Medical Ethics*. Slough, St. Paul Publications.
5. Bourne, A. *Op. cit.*
6. Smith, S. M., Hanson, R. & Noble, S. (1973) Parents of battered babies: A controlled study. *British Medical Journal* 4, 388–391.
7. Gardner, R. F. R. (1975) A new ethical approach to abortion and its implications for the euthanasia dispute. *Journal of Medical Ethics*, 1, 127–133.
8. Bowlby, J. (1965) *Child Care and Growth of Love*. Harmondsworth, Penguin Books.
9. Millard, D. W. (1971) The Abortion Decision. *British Journal of Social Work*, 1, 131.
10. Gardner, R. F. R. (1973) *Moral Dilemmas in Contraceptive Developments*. London, Christian Medical Fellowship.
11. Kluge, E.-H. W. (1975) *The Practise of Death*. Yale University Press.

Further Reading

Callahan, N. D. (1970) *Abortion: Law, Choice and Morality*. New York, Macmillan.
Church Assembly Board for Social Responsibility (1965) *Abortion in Ethical Discussion*. London, Church Information Office.
Gardner, R. F. R. (1972) *Abortion: The Personal Dilemma*. Exeter, Paternoster Press.
Noonan, J. T. (Ed.) (1970) *The Morality of Abortion: Legal and Historical Perspectives*. Harvard University Press.
O'Donovan, O. (1973) *The Christian and the Unborn Child*. Bramcote, Nottinghamshire, Grove Books.

Sex Education
Jennifer Robinson

Today, for the first time in history, 'sex' is a subject taught in schools. Sex Education has come to mean organizing graduated programmes of instruction for children and adolescents. Such teaching by its very nature cannot be purely technical for it is bound to convey an attitude. This is clearly indicated by the different names given to such courses by Education Authorities. If, for example, men and women are regarded merely as animals in a materialistic and mechanistic universe *'Sex Instruction'* suffices. If, on the other hand, they are seen as responsible and interdependent beings *'Education in Personal Relationships'* is appropriate. Those who wish to emphasize the importance of the family unit as a basis for society use the term *'Education for Marriage and Family Life'*.

The fact that there are now no generally accepted standards for sexual behaviour adds further complications to this area of human activity which is always controversial and highly emotional. Hitherto, the accepted code in the Western civilized world has been largely based on the Judaeo-Christian ethic of marriage as a relationship of equals continuing through life with premarital chastity and marital fidelity. With the decline of influence of Christian belief the emphasis has shifted towards individual freedom. At first such a change went unnoticed, for we continued to live off the legacy of the past; but, as a result of the sexual revolution which swept the Western World in the 1960s, long-standing patterns of conduct were very rapidly eroded.

Society is now in a quandary. There are, of course, those who still adhere to the former ideals, including the majority of Christians. There are many others who believe that there are valid medical, psychological and cultural reasons why sexual activity outside marriage should not be accepted as a normal way of living. But all shades of opinion exist. Some have turned to a 'situational ethic', asserting that sexual behaviour has nothing to do with reason or laws or customs, nor can we learn anything about it from the natural world or by divine revelation. Love, they say, should be the guiding principle. The criterion for what is right or wrong is what appears to be good for each individual in a given situation. Others, encouraged by the mass media with their blatantly materialistic outlook steadily pursue pleasure for its own sake regardless of any other consideration. Both of these ideas come to grief sooner or later on the rocks of human selfishness leading, as they have done, to the recent increase in promiscuity, early teenage pregnancies, venereal disease, single

72

parent families and the attempts to publicize and popularize deviational sex behaviour.

Doctors from many branches of medicine, including general practitioners, gynaecologists, psychiatrists and community physicians are involved both in formal sex education and in the counselling of young people. Before they attempt to guide others it is essential that they should be sure of their own attitude to what is right and wrong in sexual behaviour. They also need to be well acquainted with the many differing points of view on these subjects so as to be able to appreciate the intense pressures on young people today.

The Doctor's Contribution

The doctor has a special contribution to make because he can speak with authority from his knowledge and experience.

Physical Problems

1. Pregnancy in unmarried teenagers – particularly those who are very young can be damaging. Physical maturity is not reached until 18 or 19 years of age by which time the female body becomes fully equipped for child-bearing. At an earlier age difficulties in parturition or injury to immature organs may occur.

2. Sexual intercourse outside marriage is the main cause of venereal disease. Gonorrhoea, the commonest, may be difficult to detect. Although it is usually curable by antibiotics, resistant strains have recently emerged which are difficult to treat. There is a substantial risk of chronic pelvic infection and subsequent sterility – perhaps in 10% of cases – especially if the infection is unrecognized early, as it well may be. Syphilis is often inconspicuous in its early stages and so may remain unrecognized leading to the late sequel of the destructive tertiary stage. A new disease, possibly transmitted sexually and now being recognized throughout the world is that caused by the cytomegalovirus. Infection of the fetus *in utero* is an important cause of morbidity and mental retardation.[1] As with rubella, if the mother is infected early in pregnancy the child may suffer.

3. Carcinoma of the cervix is said to be six times more prevalent among women who have had several sexual partners, and particularly if coitus starts at a young age. It may take 12–15 years to develop, but is now appearing in much younger age groups than hitherto. We do not yet know how the pattern will develop as the years go by.

4. The risk of an unwanted pregnancy is always present. Even if contraceptives are used (and in casual encounters they often are not) methods such as the condom or the diaphragm carry a 15%

failure rate, while chemical methods (rarely used now) are only 75% reliable. The pill, while almost completely effective as a contraceptive, can have unpleasant side effects and the contra-indications to its use are well known. It remains to be seen what the long-term effects of long continued steroid intake will be. The use of the pill by immature girls is especially undesirable as it is known to effect normal growth. When contraceptives fail abortion may be advised. The possible complications of abor-tions are well documented. They include sterility, increase in the incidence of subsequent premature births (often associated with handicapped babies) and occasional intractable cases of mental disturbance.

Psychological Problems

These may be more serious and persistent than any physical disor-der. Adolescence is the period during which a girl becomes adjusted to her role as a woman, a wife and a mother. She gradually learns to cope with her own sexual gifts and to establish her attitudes to the demands of the opposite sex. If the pace of maturing is rushed or sexual intercourse is established too early, and outside the bond of marriage, there may be difficulties later in making secure and last-ing personal relationships in marriage. The early and too precipitate sexual experiments in adolescence multiply the possibility of psychological and sexual problems in later life. The boy is less vulnerable than the girl but he too has his problems which are all to often concealed under a cloak of apparent indifference or egotism.

Social Difficulties

There is a vital need to protect those who are vulnerable within society – the mother and her child (born or unborn). Early sexual adventures may lead to a subsequent break-up of family life and to one parent families. These in their turn tend to an increase of juvenile delinquency and the victim of child abuse may be the rejected baby of an unstable home. There is a recurring cycle of mismanagement.

The doctor needs to be well informed not only on the medical problems which may have a bearing on sex education. He needs also to be wise on the social aspects so that, when asked for advice, he knows what can be done to help.

The Role of Parents

The influence of parents on the sexual development of a child begins from the moment of birth. When a child reaches the age of five years he has already acquired many fixed sexual attitudes by unconsciously absorbing those of his parents and by observing the relationship between them.

A happy home, where parents love and respect each other and their children and where discipline is maintained, is the most important means by which children attain sexual maturity. A child is most influenced by what his parents take for granted; he learns to relate to others by watching how others do it. Clear standards of behaviour provide an essential framework of authority within which a child can flourish and develop and which he can apply to his own life as he grows up. This pattern is less easy to apply today for three main reasons.

Parental Isolation

In previous centuries large families were common and relatives lived in close proximity. Parents were not left on their own to bring up their families for they were usually surrounded by their own brothers and sisters and parents. They learned how to care for children by observing older parents. Young children copied their elder brothers and sisters and all of them grew up with a first-hand knowledge of baby and child care. There was little need for verbal or formal sex education. Today, with the isolated and truncated nuclear family such natural sex education is much less likely to occur. The problem is made more acute by the ever increasing number of one-parent families, but here a doctor's guidance on how, when and where to obtain a healthy understanding of sex may be invaluable.

Woman's Role

Woman is now being persuaded to doubt her role as wife and mother. Higher education has given her new career opportunities. The woman's liberation movements have made her question the value of marriage. Even the 1975 Sex Discrimination Act has served to emphasize the equality of man and woman in contradistinction to their complementary natures. The effect of these influences has been to confuse many – and particularly the young married woman. She may no longer be able to accept herself as a wife and mother and feelings of guilt can arise. Furthermore, marriage once the highest ambition of most girls, is considered second-best; woman, it is said, should have an occupation or career outside the home. Add to this the need in times of inflation for more money in the home to maintain living standards and the pressures on her may be irresistible. But young children need their mothers as the constant provider of love and security and consistent discipline. Older children, though less demanding physically, need some unstinted time from both mother and father.

The Effects of the Media

Through newspapers, magazines, periodicals and especially television, undesirable and unwanted influences may invade the home, undermining the word and example of parents while offering a seductive and powerful authority of their own. Often an over-emphasis on the physical glamour and pleasure of sex is linked with an encouragment to material gain and a subtle denigration of marriage.

There are, however, many advantages which alert parents can enjoy today. Sex, once a taboo subject, is now more openly discussed, enabling them to communicate more freely with their children. News reports of a lost or murdered child provide an opportunity to warn a child about strangers. A divorce may emphasize to the pre-adolescent child the misery, heartbreak and insecurity caused by the separation of father and mother and the great value of marital fidelity. Similarly the lonely plight of an unmarried mother is often ample proof to the young girl that marriage is vitally important and this further implants the ideal of premarital chastity in her mind.

Childhood Development

Babyhood

A baby starts to learn about love as soon as he emerges from the warmth and security of his mother's womb. He continues to need security and when fondled, changed, and especially when breast-fed, he unconsciously absorbs his first impressions of warm, tender, satisfying and tangible love, which he mainly associates with his mother and which strengthens his bond with her. If he is deprived of this kind of love he may find difficulty later making permanent relationships both inside and outside marriage. Lack of fondling or cuddling, which, with feeding, are among the first physical pleasures, may impair his capacity for physical sexual pleasure later on.

The Toddler

The toddler absorbs attitudes and atmosphere from those around him. He has reached the stage when 'self-love' is most obvious. He is absorbed in himself – his body in particular – and in gratifying his own wishes. This is an essential part of his development because, in order to relate to others, he must first learn to respect and value himself.

When he learns to speak he will begin to ask questions about his own body or that of a new brother or sister or of his own pregnant mother. It is the parents' attitude to these early questions, rather than the actual answers they give, that is important. By it they will either produce in their child a happy acceptance of his own body and the pleasurable feelings he associates with it, or a sense of doubt and shame, which may colour his future attitude to the physical aspects of sex.

The Pre-adolescent Child

Through this period information can be given as and when it is asked for. Discussion usually comes naturally. Both boys and girls need clear facts to prepare them for the physical and emotional changes of puberty. They also need standards and ideals to counteract the sometimes ill-timed and ill-conceived information reaching them from other sources.

By implication, as well as explicitly, it can be made clear that marriage should be a permanent relationship and that the reservation of sexual intercourse until marriage is the key to lasting happiness and personal fulfilment.

Preparing a Child for the Physical State of Puberty

The age of onset of puberty varies from nine to about fifteen years, and this variation strengthens the view that sex education is much better given at home since parents will be most aware of its imminence. If parents feel unable to give it (and many prefer not to have formal talks) they should approach their doctor, teacher or church minister for help, or obtain one of the many good books available. It is here, in particular, that the doctor should be well informed on the best books that are available both for parents and for boys and girls at different stages of development.

Girls are, usually, better prepared for puberty than boys.[2] This may be because they have a natural interest in marriage; also, parents often discuss menstruation with them and this leads on to the subjects of conception, pregnancy and birth and the limitations of the family by contraception. It is ideal that a girl (or a boy) should first hear about contraception in the context of marriage and preferably at home, as this will colour his or her whole attitude towards it.

If boys are less well prepared for puberty by their parents than girls, it may be because the father/son relationship has not developed sufficiently for them to discuss sexual subjects. Another reason may be because, unlike menstruation, nocturnal emissions and masturbation are often difficult to talk about openly. Boys who do not understand that nocturnal emissions are a normal part of their development, indicating that their sexual organs are functioning properly, are likely to be worried, upset, or even shocked when they occur.

Both boys and girls at this age need information regarding their own and each other's role in procreation. They should be aware that puberty starts at different times, that there is a normal variation in the size of breasts and other sexual organs, and that this bears no relation to their essential masculinity or femininity.

Masturbation

This habit usually passes provided too much attention is not drawn to it by unnecessary discussion. Some denounce it even though there is no evidence that it causes physical harm and any neurosis is probably associated more with guilt feelings than with the practice itself. It is probably best for parents and others to advise young people to set their minds on other pursuits and that the habit is purposeless, self-limiting and undesirable, but not to rate it higher than that. If it is persistent and pre-occupies or worries a boy, he may need medical advice.

The Adolescent

Teenagers are now usually acquainted with most of the facts of life but need help in understanding how to cope with their own emotions and how to develop their own set of ideals and principles of sexual behaviour. A girl needs to appreciate the importance of dressing and behaving modestly in order not to arouse her boyfriend sexually because it might lead on to the demand for premarital intercourse. A boy, on the other hand, should know that he develops a stronger and earlier sexual drive and hence needs to put restraint on himself. It has been said that 'a girl plays at sex for which she is not ready because fundamentally she wants love; the boy plays at love for which he is not ready because he wants sex'.

Many parents today are themselves confused about sexual standards. They need to arm themselves with clear information regarding the overwhelming advantages of premarital chastity and marital fidelity. *Sound Sex Education*, a small booklet by Dr. Margaret White (1976), provides such information in a simple and straightforward way that appeals to parents, teachers and also to young people. Others are available and the general practitioner should be a ready adviser in these matters. Ideally the school also has a part to play through parent-teacher associations and here again the doctor may be asked to help. In particular, a doctor may be able to advise when deviational sexual behaviour is discussed for he can give to parents a true perspective of the subject.

Sex Education in Schools

All that is most important and lasting in sex education takes place in the home in the setting of family life. It follows, therefore, that teaching in schools achieves its best results when guided by certain principles.

1. Partnership with parents is the ideal, obtaining their support and involving them where necessary.
2. It needs to be given in the context of marriage and family.
3. It should be graduated, bearing in mind the pupil's physical and emotional development, mental ability and religious background.
4. The content of education should, as far as possible, supplement that given at home. Objective biological facts are most appropriate in the school setting, intimate discussion may not be possible or wise.

How much Sex Education is really necessary in School?

This is a vexed question on which there is no general agreement. It is a salutary thought to remember that we have managed without it for countless centuries and there has been no obvious detriment to humanity. If it is argued that children need to have a proper understanding of human physiology there can be no disagreement. If it is asserted that they need to know about sex techniques or deviations in sexual behaviour many would disagree strongly. Even the subject of contraception needs to be introduced in the right way, at the right time and by well-disposed teachers.

There is some evidence that sex education which is ill-timed or done with the wrong motive incites to premature interest and bravado. A working party of the Royal College of Obstetricians and Gynaecologists on unplanned pregnancy chaired by Sir John Peel had this to say, 'Practically nothing is known about the effects of sex education programmes, either in regard to future health and happiness of the individual children or in relation to unplanned pregnancy. It was suggested that wrongly orientated sex education could be having a result which was the exact opposite of what it was desired to achieve, in fact it was arousing curiosity and the desire to experiment. The rapidly rising incidence of unplanned pregnancies in the young age group gives some support to this idea'.[3]

On the other hand, many parents find it difficult to discuss sexual matters with their children. There is nothing necessarily blameworthy about this, if it reflects a natural reticence. In addition, there is the problem of what to say and what words to use. Most parents recognize they need help and want their children better informed. In former times churches or clubs were more effective at this point than they are now.

Methods of Working with Parents

Several Area Health Authorities (AHAs) have recognized the need to educate parents. Meetings are arranged between parents and teachers when films are shown and problems are discussed. Sometimes teacher-parent-child evenings have been held and this has the effect of promoting communication within the family. From these have emerged playcraft clubs for very young children where parents can learn together the best ways of approaching the subject of sex. More recently, lectures and discussions have been introduced at Infant Welfare Clinics where there is a captive and interested audience.

Unfortunately co-operation between school and parents is not the general rule. A questionnaire sent to 500 head teachers showed that 75% of primary school and 50% of junior school heads thought it inappropriate to discuss sex education with parents or get their co-operation.[4] Perhaps this would be of less importance at this age if teachers and parents shared a common understanding of the place of sex and marriage in society.

Difficulties in Teaching Sex

A more fundamental problem arises when the school discusses the physical experiences of sex in total detachment from the context of marriage or of any moral norms. One reason given for doing this is the fact that today many children are without one or both natural parents and they ought not, so it is said, to be embarrassed. On the other hand, is this reason enough for confusing the majority who do have two parents?

Another reason why teaching about the facts of sex is deliberately divorced from the context of love and marriage is the wide spectrum of views held bs the teachers themselves and the lack of a common standard. Added to this there are many powerful pressure groups today actively propagating sexual licence or deviation and denigrating the institution of marriage. The schools themselves are targets for this onslaught. A leading article in the *British Medical Journal* sums it up – 'Unfortunately school sex-education has received widespread adverse publicity through the activities of a few fanatical supporters of sexual liberation: the many well-balanced lectures given by sensible experienced doctors have been ignored'.[5]

The use of visual aids may present problems. Many films and demonstrations are far too explicit. Lasting emotional damage can follow if a child is introduced too early to a pictorial exhibition for which he or she is not ready. Shock or revulsion or premature experimentation may follow. Some material shown in Youth Clubs is frankly offensive.

Secondly, care needs to be exercized in the choice of literature. The BMA, National Marriage Guidance Council and Catholic Marriage Council provide appropriately graded booklets in which sex is presented in the context of marriage and clear anatomical diagrams are used. On the other hand, some literature produced by the FPA could be classed as pornographic and is mainly concerned with the advertising and use of contraceptives.

Group teaching carries its own dangers especially when the groups are large. At any given age children vary in their physical and emotional development, mental ability, prior knowledge and social and religious background. Misunderstandings are bound to arise. False concepts take root. A form of group thinking may be imposed which itself will overawe the morally sensitive. There is a great need for small group and single sex discussions with the possibility of personal interchange between teacher and child whose confidentiality is strictly observed. If the marriage bond is not presented as the foundation for sexual activity the group pressure on the teenager to 'experiment' may become almost irresistible.

A criticism of some sex education programmes is that stress is laid on the abnormal aspects of sex. More time, for example, may be spent in discussing homosexuality than marriage and family. It is part of human nature to be more interested in the unusual and bizarre than in the normal. A skilled leader's firm hand is the obvious answer but do we have such able leaders?

Many AHAs have produced excellent programmes of health education or education in personal relationships. Regrettably, controversial, unwise or extreme views have been introduced and *integrated* into the curricula by other Authorities. It is then very difficult for parents to remove their child from such unwelcome instruction even though what many would regard as their natural rights as parents are being overruled.

Summary

Our first need is to be clear what 'sex education' is all about. It is not simply a matter of providing information to children about the facts of sexual physiology, the varieties and uses of contraceptives and some of the deviations of sexual behaviour. Rather, we are concerned to ensure that children can develop an emotional, psychological and spiritual maturity in each other's company and lay firm foundations for stable and happy relationships in marriage. If this is true then 'sex education' as it is now being propagated is far too limited a concept and is sometimes damaging in content; moreover, it should not be the monopoly interest of a few.

To achieve a balance we must agree as a nation that the right place for the physical expression of sex is within the marriage bond. Secondly, we need to reiterate again and again that attitudes to sex are absorbed within the home from infancy onwards, hence the importance of parental example. This needs to be reinforced by graded information first from parents and then from selected school teachers working in harmony to the same end. In days when sex is so much discussed and visual information is offered on a scale previously unknown in the world, careful planning of what is taught and how it is presented to young people is all the more important.

References

1. Editorial (1977) *Lancet*, **2**, 541.
2. Schofield states that one in ten boys and one in five girls can be said to have received adequate sex education. Schofield, M. (1973) *The Sexual Behaviour of Young Adults*. London, Allen Lane, p. 25.
3. *Report (1972) of a Working Party on Unplanned Pregnancy*. Chairman Sir John Peel. London, Royal College of Obstetricians and Gynaecologists, p. 83.
4. Rogers, R. P. (Ed.) (1964) *Sex Education Rationale and Reactions*. Cambridge University Press, p. 67.
5. Editorial (1973) *British Medical Journal*, **3**, 121.

Further Reading

It is very doubtful if the knowledge and wisdom needed to impart an understanding of relationships between men and women can ever be contained within the pages of books. The following have been found useful by the author and they offer some insights into the size of the problems of those who are called on to give sex education to young people.

Barclay, W. (1971) *Ethics in a Permissive Society*. London, Fontana.
Davidson, A. (1976) *The Return of Love. A contemporary Christian View of Homosexuality*. London, Intervarsity Press.
Dawkins, Julia, (1967) *A Text Book of Sex Education*. Oxford, Blackwell.
Girl's Questions Answered. Boy's Questions Answered. Both published by National Marriage Guidance Council.
Hansard, Vol. 367, No. 18. *Sex Education of Children*. London, HMSO.
Report (1964) *Venereal Disease and Young People*. London, BMA.
Rogers, R. S. (1964) *Sex Education: Rationale and Reaction*. Cambridge University Press.
Schofield, M. (1965) *Sexual Behaviour of Young People*. London, Longmans.
Schofield, M. (1973) *Sexual Behaviour of Young Adults*. London, Allen Lane.
Thielicke, H. (1964) *The Ethics of Sex*. Edinburgh, James Clarke.
White, M. (1976) *Safety and The Pill*. The Responsible Society.
White, M. (1976) *Sound Sex Education*. The Order of Christian Unity.

6

Dilemmas in the Management of Infants and Children
Janet Goodall and Ralph Evans

A child does not choose to be born. Speculating on such a choice later some would have opted themselves out of existence[1] while others with distressing handicaps would still vote in favour of life. These opposing attitudes depend on the nature of the handicap (be it physical, mental or both), the personality and intelligence of the handicapped person, and his life experience or – in other words – his *awareness*.

The ethical dilemmas at the beginning of life, however, have to be faced by others on behalf of one who, as yet, is quite *un*aware of the problems and whose personality and capacity for fortitude remain veiled. The least such a child deserves is that those who take the decisions do so responsibly, having respect not only for a particular collection of living cells, but also for the embryo person who inhabits them. Modern advances may tell us something about the cells but little about the person. Here, at the start of life, we are starkly confronted with these two aspects of medicine: 'Science deals with what is. . . . Ethics deals with what ought to be'.[2]

The Issues

The two traditional aims of medicine are the prevention of suffering and the preservation of life. When ethical dilemmas arise they usually do so because attention to the first endangers fulfilment of the second. In these dilemmas, our 'considerations about happiness and the relief of suffering need to be supplemented by sharp reminders that life is sacred whether we are happy or not. But conversely, the principle of the sacredness of life is not to be applied woodenly as if all types and qualities of human life in all circumstances ought unthinkingly to be preserved'.[3]

Whose Suffering? At the start of life it is possible for parents to suffer more keenly than a child who has never known normality. Even so, a child unaware of his handicap may suffer chronic unhappiness or the discomforts of recurrent surgery. Time may hurt rather than heal if it brings with it a hopeless awareness of permanent disability.[4]

What Kind of Life? Although we have all seen that triumph over adversity is possible, there are unbearable ills which we would not willingly inflict on others. 'Suffering . . . should be regarded, if it comes to ourselves, as an opportunity; but in the case of another we should . . . struggle with all our power to relieve him of it.'[5] Clearly, there are times when we must seem cruel to be kind, but these are not usually occasions for dispute. Before starting on controversial treatment we must have a clear idea that, in the patient's terms, the expected return is going to be worthwhile. Even if our heroic measures could save a life, we should first consider whether it would also take a hero to go on living it.

What Means?   Science can tell us the likely nature of suffering and the means available to curtail it. Ethics must decide what means justify which end. The quality of life to be preserved comes into the reckoning and so must the choice of ordinary or extraordinary means to be used in its preservation. There sometimes comes a point when what *could* be done is not what *should* be done.

The Balance   While holding firmly to the principle of the sanctity of human life, we feel it right to hold in tension the balance between the prevention or protraction of suffering on the one hand and, on the other, the worthwhile nature of the life preserved. Underlying these personal questions lies another: is it in society's interest to maintain, at great expense, a life which will in material terms make no return? It has been said that a sensitive index of any nation's level of cultural development is the provision it makes for its handicapped children.[6] In addition, we cannot know the unseen *benefits* which a society may reap by taking care of its disabled members. Although important, we agree that economic arguments should usually come second in ethical discussions.[7]

Preconception

Genetic Counselling (see also Chapter 4)

The first decision is whether a child ought ever to be conceived. Everyone is concerned to prevent birth defects and metabolic disease rather than to treat them. The birth of an affected child is often the first clue to the existing hazard, except in populations at special risk, as for instance, the Ashkenazi Jews who may carry Tay-Sachs disease, with severe mental retardation in affected children.

Once a chromosomal or genetically determined disorder has been recognized in a child, the parents must be clearly forewarned about risks to subsequent children. The geneticist, paediatrician and obstetrician should confer in the cause of accuracy and give the fullest possible information.

Genetic Risks   Medical advisers need to be up-to-date on the statistics in these matters. The overall risk of severe congenital malformation in the population is 1 in 50. In genetic terms, a risk is reckoned as high as if it is 1 in 10 or worse, and is usually 1 in 4 or 1 in 2. Parents are more likely to take on a high risk when the condition leads to an early death (e.g. Werdnig-Hoffman lower motor neurone disease), if it is treatable (Hirschsprung's disease), or if it is relatively mild (ectodermal dysplasia). Serious, advancing conditions such as pseudohypertrophic muscular dystrophy are less commonly risked. Lower risks are usually accepted unless the first child has been a great family burden, for example with spina bifida.[8] Then, even though the risk of recurrence is at least as low as 1 in 20, some parents still decide against further children.

Prenatal Problems

Prenatal Counselling

Even with responsible parents, contraception may fail. The parents' personal decision is then that of asking for and reacting to advice, but it is a professional decision as to what should be advised. If abortion is to be accepted it is important to try to define what constitutes a handicap severe enough to make life an unacceptable burden.

Prenatal Screening (see p. 44)

In certain specified problems, *amniocentesis* may turn probabilities into certainties.

Rubella in a patient whose mother is in the first trimester of pregnancy may also involve the paediatrician in prenatal screening. Although a rise in antibody is not complete proof of associated fetal infection, it is almost so.[9] If affected, a fetus may suffer a spectrum of abnormality in the cardiovascular, nervous and special sense systems. Children who previously seemed unaffected at birth may yet develop deafness or degenerative central nervous system diseases later on. The potential risk of such damage makes abortion for maternal rubella common practice. A better alternative would be to immunize pre-pubertal girls against the disease.

We see prenatal screening as a means of avoiding serious suffering to families already known to be at risk. We do not advocate its wholesale use, neither would we consider it as a determinant of fetal sex for other than medical reasons.

Perinatal Problems

Some would see no difference between fetal and neonatal life. At the extremes of viewpoint, one group regards all induced abortion as murder: the other recommends infanticide for a child found to be badly deformed at birth, especially if prenatal recognition of the deformity would have been a warrant for abortion. We believe that whatever his condition, the newborn child is now an individual, entering upon what has been described as 'the most basic right enjoyed by every human being – the right to life itself'.[10] The World Health Organization declaration of 1952 from the Expert Committee on Physically Handicapped Children also states: 'Every child regardless of his physical handicap has the right to develop to the maximum of his abilities in spite of his disablement'.[11]

Congenital Disabilities

It is often at the very beginning of life that these two 'rights' – to live and to develop – have to be considered from the viewpoint of the child himself. A baby may be born with severe disabilities which are completely treatable, partially treatable, or untreatable. We and his parents are responsible, on the child's behalf, for deciding how far we should go in our assaults. In our enthusiasm for the *surgical* conquest of physical handicaps we must beware that we are not 'developing to the maximum' a child's capacity for suffering. The quality of life that we offer must be carefully considered right at the start. 'With our team approaches ... monitoring capabilities, ventilatory support systems and intravenous hyperalimentation ... we can wind up with 'viable' children, three and four years old, well below the third percentile in height and weight, propped up on a pillow ... looking forward to another operation.'[12] Similarly, we need to consider carefully the *medical* dilemma of how vigorous we should be in our attempts at resuscitation of certain infants.

Surgically Treatable Defects

Wholly treatable?   Defects which are eminently treatable are conditions such as cleft lip or palate, Hirschsprung's disease and pyloric stenosis. They are all likely to become evident in the first few weeks of life, if not at birth. They are polygenically determined diseases, although contraception is not usually practised to avert them; there is generally no difficulty in obtaining parental consent for treatment. These conditions, once carrying a high mortality, are now likely to increase in frequency in the community as survivors produce children,[13] but this should never be a contra-indication to treatment.

Duodenal atresia is also straightforward to treat. The ethical problem arises, as not infrequently happens, when it is found to be associated with trisomy 21 anomaly (mongolism). Is it then right (or wrong) to operate and thus preserve a handicapped life? Is it wrong (or right) to allow the child to die by starvation? Neither alternative is wholly good. A similar dilemma obtains when such a severely handicapped child develops pneumonia or goes into cardiac failure, but by then parents have usually had time to form a relationship and may even urge doctors to treat. Some authors see the capacity for relationship as an overwhelming reason to operate on atresia in such an infant,[14] while others would decide to accept parental refusal for surgery.[15] 'What can reasonably be asked is that before making his decision, the doctor should inform himself fully about medical and social consequences – not only in general terms, but also in terms of the individual patient.'[16] Paediatrician, surgeon and parents should confer in such decision-making.

Wholly or partially treatable? Myelomeningocoele   This condition, in which the neural plaque is exposed, is perhaps the most difficult, and certainly the most publicized, of the partially treatable entities which confront us at birth. Here, definition of the quality of life is difficult, including as it does parameters of intelligence, mobility, continence, courage and acceptance of the child by both family and society. Because the decision is so momentous and so complex, it is more than ever necessary that it be made by more than one person. In the USA the team may include laity and clergy as well as hospital staff.[17]

In Britain, to date, the paediatrician and neurosurgeon will confer with the parents and possibly with the general practitioner. Within the team there may be a cross-section of ethical views. An amalgam of these brings the eventual decision for each particular baby. There are no blanket rules to cover each circumstance and we stress here the importance of a separate decision for each individual child. Every effort must be made to withstand legislation on this delicate issue.

Before the 1960s operation on myelomeningocoele was rare. The survival rate was 5–10% and the survivors were severely handicapped, both physically and intellectually. After a controlled trial of early surgical closure, a comprehensive programme of treatment was devised in the 1960s. The survival rate rose to 50–60%. Although some children benefited, many survived to be heavily handicapped with paraplegia, incontinence, hydrocephalus (precariously controlled) and subnormality of intellect, together with immense frustration and sometimes severe depression. Most had undergone five or six major operations in their first few years. In both personal and economic terms that cost would be high enough; the toll increases with the need to supply calipers and wheelchairs, constant medical and frequent hospital treatment plus the provision of special schools and centres for the handicapped.

In 1971, disturbed by this iatrogenic heartache and the possible misuse of resources, Lorber analysed the results of treating all comers. He isolated specific adverse criteria found at birth, which included clinically evident hydrocephalus, lower limb paralysis,

severe kyphosis and other major congenital defects.[18] Such studies
suggest that there are children who will benefit from total treatment
but, despite all efforts, there are others who will have little chance of
a satisfying life. On this evidence, many units are now practising a
policy of selection for surgery. Some children are not being submitted
to early surgery and some who develop life-threatening complications, such as ventriculitis, are not receiving treatment.

Naturally, there are those who disagree with this policy and take
the view that to withold antibiotics is negligence.[19, 20] Certainly it is
easier to decide to treat every child, as both medical and nursing staff
find an inactive policy runs counter to their training. It is also true
that to treat every child may initially help the parents. However, the
first person to be considered in every such decision is the child
himself. When we are assessing the future of a small, crippled, newborn baby we must face the probability of the child's surviving to
become a severely handicapped individual with an almost superhu-
man burden to bear. We must consider the questions – Whose suffering? What means and to which end? What kind of life? . . . It is
possible to solve our own problems by perpetuating in the life of
another an even greater one. While we fully support the concept of
reverence for human life, we clearly distinguish between *cure* – or
attempt at it – and *care*. There is again a difference between care
which may be deemed ordinary and that which, in certain circumstances, could be extraordinary.

If we cannot cure, treatment in any terminal illness should be
directed towards comfort. This holds in the terminal stages of
leukaemia, for example, as well as in the area under discussion. Few
would dispute that to deny food when requested is to deny care. Yet to
withhold antibiotics can be to show true care, if to give them would
prolong dying rather than enrich living. To give sedatives or analgesics to relieve distress is also part of care, although we would be
against offering a deliberately lethal dose.

Having decided not to prolong suffering we must still consider the
quality of the baby's life even if it is to be short. Ordinary care of any
baby means to provide food and rest, comfort and love, and these can
all be offered to a child who has not been selected for surgery. Parents
are welcome to participate in this management. Given the chance –
and also given the support – many parents accept such involvement
and some even take the child home.[21] Involving themselves thus, they
recognize the baby's increasing weakness and can prepare themselves for bereavement when it comes, usually in weeks or months.
To allow this anticipatory grief is painful to both parents and professionals and takes more time and involvement by senior staff than
would the avoidance of any such contact. However, it produces
immediate comfort for the child and ultimate consolation to the
parents when it can be done. To bid them forget that they ever had
this baby and to deny further contact is to deprive both child and

parents. It would not be compassionate to force such involvement, but parents should be given this option, and many take it. Occasionally, a child who was initially thought to be unsuitable for surgery survives and thrives. Even after two or three months operation can still be offered. As the child was already heavily handicapped, the delay will not have made matters worse.

Medically Treatable Disease

Wholly treatable?   Enzyme defects Phenylketonuria typifies a group of diseases which, untreated, produces brain damage. Its incidence in the West is 1 in 10,000. Early recognition and dietary treatment (involving family co-operation) make it possible for the child to grow up intellectually normal. The high cost of screening and diet must be balanced against that of providing care for untreated children; for phenylketonuria this is probably a cost effective exercise.[22] However, universal screening for other treatable disease such as galacto-saemia, although desirable, is not yet practical in economic terms. To screen for *un*treatable disease, such as muscular dystrophy, is an ideal which could help in genetic counselling and give a truer aware-ness of the disease distribution. On economic grounds it is so far unjustified on a universal scale, although it can be valuable in affected families.

Wholly or partially treatable?   Intensive neonatal care. Enthusiastic resuscitation of infants with perinatal anoxia, and improved care for small preterm babies has resulted in an overall decline in mortality during the last two decades. Even so, a decision has to be made whether the routine use of extraordinary means of support (such as mechanical ventilation) is justified for all scarcely viable babies. Such lives may prove to have been prolonged at the cost of intellect and independence. In one series, 10% of survivors of mechanical ventilation had moderate to severe neurological sequelae. Even so, the authors also described a reduction in the incidence of spastic diplegia since the institution of intense neonatal care in the mid 1960s, although they were instead seeing children with other kinds of cerebral damage, who had presumably survived as a result of ventila-tion.[23]

We urgently need practical guidelines before extraordinary means become universally accepted as ordinary ones. Such evidence is slowly accruing. Efforts are being made to analyse what kind of respiratory support should be offered to which kind of baby, this being the neonatologist's dilemma.

(a) *Intermittent positive pressure ventilation* (IPPV) *Severe birth asphyxia* Faced with an apparent stillbirth, a junior doctor may fear to resuscitate lest he preserves a 'vegetable' life. There are now several encouraging reports following up such infants who have survived if given IPPV promptly, even after having asphyxia severe enough to give an Apgar score of 0 at one minute and less than 4 at 5 minutes. In their series, Thomson *et al*. have deduced that 'the quality of life enjoyed by the large majority (93%) of the survivors was such as to justify a positive approach to the resuscitation of very severely asphyxiated neonates'.[24]

The pathophysiological explanation for this is that the brain stem in the newborn infant is selectively more vulnerable to asphyxia than the relatively under-developed cortex: granted brain stem survival, we may expect little cortical damage.[25]

Persistent apnoea after delivery When an infant does not respond to IPPV, the doctor's next problem is, 'How long to keep trying?' Steiner and Neligan have shown that if the heart is restored at birth, but spontaneous respiration is not then established within half an hour, the prognosis is very poor, with gross handicap in the children who survive.[26] Half an hour would thus seem an appropriate time to strive, and, if there is no response by then, to stop.

(b) *Continuous positive airway pressure* (CPAP)   This is provided for the spontaneously breathing infant to increase the distending pressure of the lungs. In many infants this is adequate to maintain satisfactory levels of oxygen. Anxiety may arise when a scarcely viable infant does not respond and remains hypoxic. Should mechanical ventilation be considered? Some experienced workers would avoid it in babies of less than 1500 g while others would be ready to ventilate infants of less than 1000 g.[27] Clearly long-term follow-up is needed before we know how truly successful are the survivals claimed.

(c) *Mechanical ventilation*   Recurrent apnoeic attacks commonly occur in the survivors of severe perinatal asphyxia, in small preterm infants or in babies who are ill. Ethical considerations apart, in all these infants the cause for apnoea or hypoxia must be clarified before considering continuous ventilation. Thus, it would not cure underlying septicaemia, hypoglycaemia or congenital heart disease. IPPV may give time to clarify and treat such basic problems and, in emergencies, must clearly be given. The question remains as to which babies should eventually go on to a mechanical ventilator.

The 'cerebral' baby Infants resuscitated after severe asphyxia may, hours later, have symptoms suggestive of disturbed cerebral metabolism. Although these are not necessarily indicative of permanent brain damage, there is a natural hesitancy to offer such infants mechanical ventilatory support. The presence of large retinal haemorrhages or of blood in the cerebrospinal fluid are both suggestive of organic brain damage rather than of temporary upset following anoxia and are clearly adverse findings.

In order to clarify which babies should be helped, Brown *et al*. have described seven clinical signs which can be of prognostic significance, namely; apnoeic or cyanotic attacks, feeding difficulties necessitating tube feeds, apathy, convulsions, hypothermia, a cerebral cry and persistent vomiting. In their series no child with only one of these criteria died, but with five or more symptoms 90% of babies died or had severely residual handicap. If *tone* alone were studied, prolonged hypotonia carried a bad prognosis while infants with normal tone after cerebral anoxia grew up without significant handicap.[28] These findings offer ways of assessing likely prognosis in a 'cerebral' baby, which may help to be decisive in the proposed use of mechanical ventilation. Other writers have shown that repeated convulsions following asphyxia carry a bad prognostic index and are commoner in preterm infants.[29]

Hyaline membrane disease There is now evidence to show that the *early* use of CPAP in infants with hyaline membrane disease may modify the course of the disease and avoid the need for mechanical ventilation.[30] Persistent hypoxia or apnoea requiring more than 10 minutes of hand ventilation are taken as indications for mechanical ventilation.

When making such decisions on a basis of weight, it must be remembered that Asian and African babies have a smaller average birth weight than Caucasians. Also, every paediatrician recognizes a great variation in the apparent innate strength of small babies. The figures quoted on 'cerebral' babies and ventilated babies result from work on infants who were in difficulties for a variety of reasons. Clearly, any baby must again be judged on individual grounds, but if deemed treatable the exercise must be pursued wholeheartedly and competently. If local conditions do not allow this, the child should be transferred to a special unit. Long term follow up will clarify whether present thinking needs further modification.

A doctor looking after the newborn must learn *the signs of cerebral death* and be prepared to stop efforts when these are found. They include terminal gasping or absent respirations, no eye movements or pupillary response, absent tone (although small infants may stiffen) and absent reflexes.[31] To prolong ventilation of a dead baby is to prolong anxiety for the parents.

Partially treatable disease? Cystic fibrosis (One in 2000 births among Caucasians) may be suspected at birth, but there is yet little evidence that early diagnosis greatly improves the prognosis. Reliable routine screening is not yet available. Meconium ileus, causing gut obstruction in the newborn, may be considered a death sentence, but most surgeons will still operate without question. The disease advances with variable severity and at unpredictable rates. Supportive treatment may give years of worthwhile life: it must always include support to parents, who may well realise that they are living with approaching death.

Informed – and Educated – Consent

To tell is not necessarily to explain, even though it should be. As parental consent for therapeutic procedures has to be granted (or withheld), it is important that such consent is both informed and instructed.[32, 33] It must never be suggested, for instance, that a child with spina bifida can be *cured* by surgery or that once his duodenal atresia is corrected a mongol child will be normal. Tragic disappointments have been in store for many parents to whom the issues were not made clear at the start. The obvious difficulty is that in the shock and distress of the immediate postnatal period, they are often in no fit state to see the problem objectively. They often admit a trustful dependence on their medical advisers which must be responsibly honoured. A doctor should be aware that his judgment can be swayed by feelings of prejudice which may be irrelevant to the main issue. Any action which is judged to be in the child's best interest is crucial and should be explained to the parents with sensitivity and clarity. It helps them to realize that this is a composite view, formed after discussion between appropriate experts as well as with themselves.

Consent for Research (see p. 148)

The conclusions concerning the management of spina bifida were reached by a retrospective survey. There are areas where comparative studies of controlled series would be valuable for prospective study, but: 'In the strict meaning of the law parents and guardians of minors cannot give consent on their behalf to any procedures which have no particular benefit to them and which may carry some risk of harm'.[34] Views differ as to whether this dictum should be changed,[35, 36] but as it stands it constitutes an ethical dilemma. While allowing comparisons between accepted methods of treatment it inhibits non-therapeutic research on children and denies them the benefits of new diagnostic methods of treatment which could have been discovered thereby.

In practice it is recommended that any procedures not in the ordinary course of medical care should have specific parental consent and no new therapeutic procedures should be applied to children until the principles have been tested by animal experiments.[37]

'Under no circumstances is a doctor permitted to do anything that would weaken the physical and mental resistance of a human being except from strictly therapeutic or prophylactic indications imposed in the interest of his patient.' (World Medical Association 1949). It would seem permissible to take for research purposes a specimen of cord blood, or an extra aliquot of blood, when it was necessary to take a specimen for the child's benefit. At the other end of the spectrum, studies have taken place on children which some consider should never have been countenanced.[38, 39]

Consent for Investigation

Some investigations are hazardous. They should only be ordered in the patient's interest, not merely for the doctor's interest. Parents should be clearly informed before major procedures are carried out on a child and their agreement obtained.

Court Orders

Refusal of Treatment

During treatment there may be times when the doctor's opinion about what is the right course of action clashes with that of the parents. The doctor advises treatment and the parents – through misunderstanding, religious conviction or emotional disturbance – refuse to agree to it. A dispassionate medical opinion should be offered. If it is then agreed that the proposed action must be taken, the child can be made a ward of court and the surgery, transfusion, or other treatment given with official authorization. This makes for problems in the child's aftercare and it is better if the matter can be calmly reviewed with the parents, and their voluntary agreement sought. Even without a court order any legal action will be likely to fail if brought against a doctor who has clearly acted in the child's interests (Medical Defence Union).

Non-accidental Injury

The commoner use of court orders is to protect a child thought to be at risk from either severe neglect or of non-accidental injury. It has been increasingly recognized over the last ten years that injuries sustained by young children may have been deliberately inflicted by parents or child minders. Local Health Authorities have evolved procedures for managing the condition and doctors are commonly involved, either as the patient's first contact or because the Social Services, for example, need a medical opinion.[40] However the patient presents, the parents have to be questioned, and, if the explanations offered are incompatible with the injuries, a case conference has to be arranged.

This kind of responsibility is stressful for all concerned. Medical consultation is usually based on mutual trust, but here it can arouse mutual suspicion. Inference of parental guilt may produce aggression. Exposure of parental guilt strains medical confidentiality. The doctor is in an area foreign to his training: tension mounts if he finds himself in conference with police anxious to convict the parents or social workers anxious to remove the child. The protection of the child is, of course, paramount and most parents – even if with reluctance or shame – will accept that information given to the doctor must, in these circumstances, be shared with others. (The writers feel strongly, though, that just as a wife is exempt from testifying against her husband, so evidence from a child about his parents should not be used in court). While a clear understanding must be sought about the nature of the child's injuries, the personality of the parents and the state of the home, all those who confer must also remember the emotional needs of children. It may be thought that by removing a child from home 'into care' he is protected from injury, but sometimes little thought is given to the fact that this move may cause more hurt to a child's bewildered mind than ever was done to his body.

At present, it is easy to remove a child from home on a place of safety order, but a supervision order has to wait for a court hearing. This may take weeks to arrange, and meantime the child has to be kept out of his immediate family. Whereas it is right to seek to avoid tragedy, it is wrong to send a child into exile without being as sure as we can that his injuries were genuinely non-accidental. Otherwise, in the very attitude of care, we may act with cruelty. In some areas, there is now an encouraging trend to drop a place of safety order which was taken out in a crisis if the parents will agree to allow continuing supervision by the Social Services.

Unhappily, there are many families in which there is no doubt that the child has been neglected or deliberately hurt. The decision of the court in such cases has usually been to choose the supposedly lesser of two evils and to remove the child. In many of these cases, to treat the family would be both a protection and a remedy for the child. Family care centres are expensive, but have been shown to be effective in the promotion of family health.[41] If a cycle of deprivation can thereby be avoided this kind of management would, in the long term, be an economy when balanced against the cost of years of residential care for deprived children.

Adoption

For similar reasons, abrupt removal from natural or foster parents is, to a child who has had time to become attached to them, an inexplicable bereavement. Adoption needs to be arranged as early as possible so that strong long-lasting emotional bonds may be developed with the new parents. It has, however, been traditional to be as sure as possible that a child is normal before finalizing adoption, but as fostering is the usual compromise during the waiting period, bonding is repeatedly disrupted. This must cause major upsets in the child's emotional security whatever the ultimate judgment on his physical state. Adoption agencies must be helped to understand this, for if adopting parents had a full understanding of the underlying problems for the child many would opt for early adoption despite any implicit risk.

Adoption of handicapped children is becoming commoner. This may produce conflicts between the ideal of early placement and the delay before a confident prognosis can be offered. Medical examinations of children for adoption should be performed by experts; the same examiner should perform both the initial and the three month examinations whenever possible. The cardinal consideration in adoption should be the welfare of the child and it should not be arranged in the hope of resolving marital difficulties or any other remote problems in the parent.

Although most children settle happily into loving homes, various difficulties may arise after adoption. Some, such as stealing and aggression require understanding rather than punishment, for they are emotional rather than moral aberrations. We can avoid suffering for both the adopted child and his parents by anticipating and explaining such problems.

Children at Risk

Babies with a potential handicap are often identified at birth because of damaging circumstances such as anoxia and dysmaturity. It is now established that we can also identify some children who are at risk either of *non-accidental injury* or *cot-death*. There is now evidence that the former include babies who were in special care baby units.[42] An index of suspicion for the latter is that appointments to infant follow-up clinics are not kept.[43] Any failed appointee who is illegitimate, preterm and whose teenage mother was careless about attendance at antenatal clinic fulfils criteria known to be adverse to the child's welfare.

Workers in Sheffield are elaborating a scoring system, based on factors noted at birth and at one month of age, by which infants at risk of unexpected death may be identified.[44] The provision of increased health visitor care to babies known to be at risk has already resulted in a drop in unexpected deaths in Sheffield infants. Unfortunately, their criteria do not apply universally; nevertheless, this work provides a model for the identification and care of infants at risk elsewhere.

In the light of such knowledge we are morally wrong to cross off our clinic list any child known to fall into the 'at risk' categories, or who fails to attend. Arrangements should be made to have the care taken to the home while leaving the door open for review in clinic. In economic terms alone, our clinics expend a lot of time and money on those who need least supervision.[45]

Accidental Injury

Childhood accidents constitute the largest single cause of death between the ages of 1 and 15, causing more deaths than the two next commonest causes combined. They have consistently headed this list of causes of death for the past twenty-five years or more and until recently there has been no sign of a reduction in the total numbers.[46] Many of these accidents occur because children are having to live in a world designed for adults by adults. Since 1961, organizations such as the Medical Commission on Accident Prevention have been analysing modes of accident causation and suggesting methods of accident prevention. As the facts emerge, we have a moral responsibility to influence architects, motorists, packagers of drugs and any other body whose activities are likely to put children at risk.

Hospital Admission

Any child under the age of three years is likely to suffer when undergoing protracted separation from his mother or loved mother-substitute. This can happen during a hospital admission. Despite a father's importance in providing emotional security, his close presence is usually less vital to the child's daily comfort so that it is usually the mother to whom the paediatric unit will offer accommodation during a child's illness. There are still unenlightened areas where a child may be admitted alone to an adult ward, with restricted visiting times. Sometimes isolation in a cubicle has to happen, but it should not be unnecessarily prolonged. Such experiences may produce protracted emotional disturbances which could largely be avoided by a little thought and by encouragement of the mother's involvement. It is for these reasons that most paediatricians practise out-patient rather than in-patient care whenever possible.

The Disturbed Child

A large percentage of paediatric out-patient attenders come with emotional problems disguised as physical disorders. A child's basic emotional needs have been described as affection – offered in a sustained loving relationship with parents – personal significance within a caring family group, scope for self expression, and reasonable, consistent discipline.[47] An imbalance between needs felt and needs met is emotionally disturbing. To prevent emotional suffering as well as to alleviate physical symptoms we need to spend time and interest in unravelling these problems. It is far easier, but not always justified, to prescribe tranquillizers or antidepressants.

The Disabled Child

If we are to improve the quality of life for handicapped children we must attend to more than their physical needs. It is possible for them both to feel handicapped through and through and to use their disability as a means of getting their own way. It should be part of our care to inspire as robust and independent a spirit as possible even where the body is frail and helpless; this attitude must also be communicated to the parents and teachers. Particular help will be needed at times of emotional crisis such as on entering and leaving school or when disability suddenly seems overwhelming for other reasons.

Iatrogenic Disease

In our attempts to prevent suffering, it is tragic that sometimes we actually promote it. For example, small neonates may be threatened with kernicterus if given sulphonomides or with retrolental fibroplasia if nursed in too high an oxygen concentration. Later in life, high steroid dosage may cause stunting or cyclophosphamide induce sterility. Perhaps more avoidable problems may arise by failing to let parents know that a child has been on steroids or has been given BCG. An unexpected collapse or a surprisingly positive Heaf test would quickly be explained on the production of the appropriate card, although all too often this has not been given. Some children who sustained brain damage following immunization might have been normal had their medical practitioner taken note of existing contra-indications to pertussis vaccine.[48]

These are but a few examples of iatrogenic disease: some are unavoidable, but many need never happen given a careful and thoughtful doctor. These qualities form part of our moral obligation to all patients.

The prime factor necessary in all the above circumstances is recognition that the problems exist. It is possible for us to be so engrossed in the conquest of physical disability that we ourselves are guilty of inflicting emotional suffering, even at the very beginning of life. We may also add to physical suffering by thoughtlessness. Genetic counselling, neonatal surgery and some of the larger ethical dilemmas are much publicized but the less obvious problems are with us every day.

The World's Children

A study of ethical problems in paediatrics would be incomplete without mentioning the imbalance in care between the children of developed and developing countries.

On a world scale most paediatric illness is preventable, but even more so in the developing countries. Here, medical services need to direct their care with this in mind, building fewer prestigious hospitals and supporting more immunization programmes. 'Although three-quarters of the population in most countries in the tropics and sub-tropics live in rural areas, three-quarters of the spending on medical care is in urban areas, and also three-quarters of the doctors live there.[49]

Paediatricians in the developed world should also question whether it is right to spend time, money and resources on esoteric investigations when millions of the world's children are at special risk of death or deprivation. Ninety per cent of the world's expenditure on health care goes to only ten per cent of the world's population. This fact makes the question about suffering, quality of life and ordinary means of care take on a greater poignancy.

References

1. Engelhardt, H. T. (1973) Euthanasia and children. *Journal of Paediatrics*; Book of Job, **10**, 18, 19.
2. Fletcher, J. (1971) Ethical aspects of genetic controls. *New England Journal of Medicine*, **285**, 776.
3. Report (1975) Ethics of selective treatment of spina bifida. *Lancet*, **1**, 85.
4. Dorner, S. (1976) Adolescents with spina bifida. *Archives of Disease in Childhood*, **51**, 439.
5. Gollancz, V. (1969) *My Dear Timothy*. Harmondsworth, Penguin Books.
6. *British Medical Journal* (1968) **2**, 573.
7. Hatcher, G. (1973) Severely malformed children. Economic grounds no criteria. *British Medical Journal*, **2**, 284.
8. Bundey, S. (1975) Genetic counselling and some ethical aspects. *In the Service of Medicine*, **21**, 15.
9. Dudgeon, J. A. (1976) Infective causes of human malformations. *British Medical Bulletin*, **32**, 77.
10. McCormick, R. A. (1974) To save or let die. *Journal of the American Medical Association*, **229**, 172.
11. WHO (1952) Technical report series, No. 58. Geneva, WHO.
12. Shaw, A. (1973) Dilemmas of "informed" consent in children. *New England Journal of Medicine*, **289**, 885.
13. Carter, C. O. (1976) Genetics of common single malformations. *British Medical Bulletin*, **32**, 21.
14. McCormick. *Op. cit.*
15. Shaw. *Op. cit.*
16. Richards, I. D. G. (1973) Quality of life: with special reference to paediatrics. *In the Service of Medicine*, **19**, 5.
17. Duff, R. S. & Campbell, A. G. M. (1973) Moral and ethical dilemmas in the special care nursery. *New England Journal of Medicine*, **289**, 890.
18. Lorber, J. (1971) Results of treatment of myelomeningocele. *Developmental Medicine and Child Neurology*, **13**, 279.
19. Zachary, R. B. (1968) Ethical and social aspects of treatment of spina bifida. *Lancet*, **2**, 274.
20. Zachary, R. B. (1977) Life with spina bifida. *British Medical Journal*, **2**, 1460.

21. Melton, J. (1978) Life with spina bifida. *British Medical Journal*, 1, 47.
22. Komrower, G. M. (1974) The philosophy and practice of screening for inherited diseases. *Paediatrics*, 53, 182.
23. Marriage, J. K. & Davies, P. A. (1977) Neurological sequelae in children surviving mechanical ventilation in the neonatal period. *Archives of Disease in Childhood*, 52, 176.
24. Thomson, A. J., Searle, M. & Russell, G. (1977) Quality of survival after severe birth asphyxia. *Archives of Disease in Childhood*, 52, 620.
25. Hull, D. (Ed.) (1976) *Recent Advances in Paediatrics* 5, chapter 2. Edinburgh, Churchill Livingstone.
26. Steiner, H. & Neligan, G. (1975) Perinatal cardiac arrest. *Archives of Disease in Childhood*, 50, 696.
27. Hull, D. *Op. cit.*, chapter 4.
28. Brown, J. K., Purvis, R. J., Forfar, J. O. & Cockburn, F. (1974) Neurological aspects of perinatal asphyxia. *Developmental Medicine and Child Neurology*, 16, 567.
29. Marriage & Davies. *Op. cit.*
30. Krouskop, R. W., Brown, E. G. & Sweet, A. Y. (1975) The early use of continuous CPAP in the treatment of idiopathic respiratory distress syndrome. *Journal of Pediatrics*, 87, 263.
31. Hull, D. *Op. cit.*, chapter 3.
32. Shaw, (1973) *Op. cit.*
33. Ingelfinger, F. J. (1972) Informed (but uneducated) consent. *New England Journal of Medicine*, 287, 465.
34. Franklin, A. W., Porter, A. M. W., & Raine, D. N. (1973) Research investigations on children. *British Medical Journal*, 2, 402.
35. Porter, A. M. W. (1973) Minors and medical experiments. *British Medical Journal*, 1, 46.
36. Hubble, D. (1973) Minors and medical experiments. *British Medical Journal*, 1, 171.
37. Editorial (1967) Treatment – Research – Experiment? *Archives of Disease in Childhood*, 42, 109.
38. Beecher, H. K. (1966) Ethics and clinical research. *New England Journal of Medicine*, 274, 1354.
39. Editorial (1968) Ethics in research. *British Journal of Hospital Medicine*, 2, 759.
40. Arthur, L. J. H., Moncrieff, W. M., Milburn, W. *et al.* (1976) Non-accidental injury in children: what we do in Derby. *British Medical Journal*, 1, 1363.
41. Lynch, M. *et al.* (1975) Family unit in a children's psychiatric hospital. *British Medical Journal*, 2, 127.
42. Lynch, M. A. (1975) Ill health and child abuse. *Lancet*, 2, 317.
43. Protestos, C. D. *et al.* (1973) Obstetric and perinatal histories of children who died unexpectedly (cot death) *Archives of Disease in Childhood*, 48, 835.
44. Carpenter, R. G., Gardner, A., McWeeny, P. M. & Emery, J. L. (1977) Multistage scoring system for identifying infants at risk of unexpected death. *Archives of Disease in Childhood*, 52, 606.
45. Zinkin, P. M., Cox, C. A. (1976) Child health clinics and inverse care laws. *British Medical Journal*, 2, 411.
46. Jackson, R. H. (Ed.) (1977) *Children, the Environment and Accidents*. London, Pitman Medical Publications.

47. Pemberton, P. (1974) *Childhood Disorders: a Psychosomatic Approach.*
    London, Crosby, Lockwood and Staples.
48. DHSS (1977) Whooping cough vaccine. London, HMSO.
49. Morley, D. (1973) *Paediatric priorities in the developing world.* London,
    Butterworth.

Further Reading

Adoption of Children (1970) Working Paper. London, HMSO.
Burton, L. (Ed.) (1974) *Care of the Child facing Death*: London, Routledge and
    Keegan Paul.
Court, D. (Ed.) (1976) Report of the Committee on Child Health Services.
    Volumes 1 and 11. London, HMSO.
Court, D., Jackson, A. (Eds.) (1973) *Paediatrics in the Seventies: Developing
    the Child Health Services.* London, Oxford University Press.
Franklin, A. W. (1976) *Pastoral Paediatrics*: London, Pitman Medical.
Freeman, J. M. (1974) *Practical Management of Meningomyelocele*: New
    York, University Park Press.
Illingworth, R. S. (1974) Some ethical problems in Paediatrics: Modern
    trends in paediatrics 4 (Ed. Apley, J.) Chapter 13. London, Butterworth.
Lubchenko, L. (1976) *The high risk infant.* Phildadelphia & London, W. B.
    Saunders.
Oppe and Woodford (Eds.) (1977) *Early Management of Handicapping Disor-
    ders*: Amsterdam, IRMMH. Reviews of Research and Practice 19.
Sheridan, Mary D. *The Handicapped Child in His Home*: London, N.C.H.

7

Decisions About Dying and Death
Robert Twycross

We live in a society which has attempted to outlaw death. Like 'sex' a hundred years ago, it is something one does not talk about. Factors such as increased safety at work, advances in preventive and curative medicine, and lack of involvement in a major war for thirty years have removed death from normal family life. The average family can now expect some twenty years of freedom from death in its immediate circle. In such circumstances it is not surprising that most of us expect to live to ripe old age. Death is dismissed from conscious thought and forms no part of our philosophy of life. We feel uneasy in the face of approaching death, and tend to withdraw from the one who needs our continued presence and companionship; supportive sympathy gives way to the paralysis of pity and we stand back appalled at the progressive deterioration of friend or loved one. Revulsion evokes an unspoken cry to end it all, which, in some cases, becomes crystallized into a demand for 'euthanasia'.

Euthanasia

The word euthanasia is derived from two Greek words, *eu* and *thanatos*, which together means without suffering. Since the foundation of the Euthanasia Society forty years ago, the word has, however, taken on a narrower meaning – the administration of a drug deliberately and specifically to accelerate death in order to end suffering. Euthanasia can either be voluntary or compulsory. Voluntary euthanasia, requested by the sufferer, has also been described as suicide by proxy or homicide by request. Compulsory euthanasia implies a decision by society to end the life of a sufferer who cannot signify volition, for example, the severely handicapped infant and the demented.

The Legal Position

In no country is either form of euthanasia legal. English law regards the killing of a human being as *prima facie* wrong and an event which requires investigation. The law does, however, regard some types of killing as more serious than others and this is reflected in the number of different offences concerned with killing which the law recognizes: murder, manslaughter, killing by dangerous driving, complicity in suicide and so on. Murder is defined as the unlawful killing of a human being with malice aforethought, express or

101

implied.[1] Manslaughter is defined in the same way but with the omission of the words *with malice aforethought, express or implied*. Whereas murder carries a mandatory sentence of life imprisonment, the penalty for manslaughter can range from an absolute discharge to imprisonment for life. At first sight it might seem that voluntary euthanasia falls within the definition of manslaughter, rather than that of murder, in as much as compassion and not malice is the motivation. The law, however, holds that intentional killing is always malicious by definition, that is, against the best interests of both the individual and society. At the present time, therefore, English law regards death acceleration as murder, whatever the motive.

Moreover, the European Convention of Human Rights in 1953 stated, in Section 1 of Article 2, 'Everyone's right to live shall be protected by law. No one shall deprive of life intentionally save in the execution of a sentence of a court following conviction of a crime for which this penalty is provided by law'. The United Kingdom was, and still is, a signatory to the convention. Earlier, in 1950, the World Medical Association declared that voluntary euthanasia is contrary to the spirit of the Declaration of Geneva and, therefore, unethical. This was endorsed by national medical associations throughout the world.

Herein lies the ethical problem. Are there circumstances in which euthanasia might, after all, be justifiable. If so, when and why? Unfortunately, many of those who seek to make euthanasia legal fail to distinguish between deliberate death acceleration and related problems, such as adequate pain relief, 'letting nature take its course', and stopping artificial ventilation, which the doctor faces when death appears inevitable in one of his patients. As a result, discussion is bedevilled by confusion arising from lack of definition.

Parliamentary Debate

In 1931, Dr. Killick Millard, president of the Society of Medical Officers of Health, asserted that 'vast numbers of human beings are doomed to end their earthly existence by a lingering, painful and often agonizing form of death'. Voluntary euthanasia should, he said, be made legal for adults suffering from an 'incurable, fatal, painful disease'.[2] Millard subsequently founded the Euthanasia Society in 1935. Its aim was:

'to create a public opinion favourable to the view that an adult person suffering from a fatal illness, for which no cure is known should be entitled by law to the mercy of a painless death if and when that is his expressed wish: and to promote this legislation'.

Since then, two Voluntary Euthanasia Bills have been presented to Parliament in the United Kingdom: both were defeated. In 1936, the situation envisaged was one in which the doctor could no longer control pain and was therefore faced with the choice of ending the patient's life or failing to relieve pain. The 1969 Bill provided that the patient or prospective patient should be able to sign in advance a declaration requesting the administration of euthanasia if he was believed to be suffering from 'a serious physical illness or impairment reasonably thought in the patient's case to be incurable and expected to cause him severe distress and render him incapable of rational existence'. In the later Bill, the requirement that the condition be fatal was omitted and the words 'incapable of rational existence' added. These modifications would have allowed a considerable extension of the range of cases eligible for euthanasia and, theoretically, could have included senile dementia and certain forms of chronic mental illness.

A third Bill to 'enlarge and declare the rights of patients to be delivered from incurable suffering' was introduced in the House of Lords in 1973.[3] It sought to establish the incurable patient's right to full relief from pain and physical distress, to remove the stigma of suicide should such a patient decide to end his life, and to give legal status to a person's written wish not to have life-sustaining treatment should he subsequently suffer from irreversible brain damage or degeneration. The Bill, defeated by 85 votes to 23, appeared to be based on two premises: that terminal pain cannot be relieved and a doctor must preserve life 'at all costs'.

Passive Euthanasia

This term has been used increasingly in recent years. It means 'letting nature take its course' instead of applying medical treatment intended to lengthen the lives of the incurably sick. As it does not involve deliberate death acceleration it should not be described as euthanasia. Moreover, its use derives from a failure to distinguish between aims of acute medicine and terminal care. Priorities change when a patient is expected to die within a few weeks or months; the primary aim is then not to preserve life but to make the life that remains as comfortable and as meaningful as possible. It has been said that the ethical justification for 'letting nature take its course' relies on the doctrine of 'acts and omissions',[4] which states that, in certain situations, failure to perform an act (e.g. prescribe an antibiotic for a patient with terminal cancer who develops pneumonia) is less bad than performing a different act (e.g. administering a lethal overdose) which has identical predictable consequences; in other words, it is more reprehensible to kill someone than to allow a person to die.

This doctrine is, however, irrelevant in the present context, and, as stated, is based on a naive understanding of clinical realities. Since death is inevitable for all of us, a doctor is bound ultimately to 'let nature take its course'. Moreover, acute and terminal illness are different patho-physiological entities. In the former, provided the patient survives the initial crisis, recovery is brought about largely by natural forces of healing; in the latter, these forces become progressively less effective as physical dissolution proceeds. In practice, therefore, the argument revolves round the question of *effective interference* and not the doctrine of 'acts and omissions'. Thus, what is appropriate in one situation may be inappropriate in the other. Gastric tubes, intravenous infusions, antibiotics, respirators and cardiac resuscitation, for example, are primarily supportive measures for use in acute illness to assist a patient through a critical period towards recovery of health. To use such measures in the terminally ill, with no expectancy of a return to health, is generally inappropriate and is therefore, by definition, bad medicine.

Since the days of Hippocrates, doctors have undertaken never to destroy life deliberately, that is, they will endeavour to sustain life when, *from a biological point of view*, it is sustainable. A doctor has no legal, moral or ethical obligation to use drugs, techniques or apparatus if their use can be described as prolonging the process of dying. He does not have a duty to preserve life at all costs. For example, when pneumonia supervenes in terminal cancer, morphine and hyoscine are commonly prescribed to quieten the cough and reduce troublesome secretions; antibiotics are inappropriate in this situation. If, however, the distinction between acute and terminal illness is ignored, the situation will not be assessed in terms of what is biologically appropriate (and therefore in the patient's best interest) but will be seen as a question of 'to treat or not to treat?'. A failure to resolve what appears to be an ethical dilemma commonly results in additional, unnecessary suffering for the patient.

Voluntary Euthanasia

The case for voluntary euthanasia depends ultimately upon the acceptance of the principle that man, when incurably or terminally ill, has the right to decide how much suffering he is prepared to accept and, when that limit is reached, he has 'a right to die', meaning a right to have death hastened deliberately. It follows that the case against voluntary euthanasia depends ultimately on the denial of the existence of such a right – a denial which has been argued on religious, moral and practical grounds. The present legal position stems from these more fundamental considerations.

Religious Considerations

In Britain, the religious argument will, generally, be from the Christian point of view. This is based on the belief not, as is sometimes stated, that life has an absolute value but that the disposal of life is in God's hands. In other words, man himself is viewed as having no absolute control over life, but as holding it in trust. Also, no one has the right to take innocent life.[5] This principle derives immediately from the fact that God is the Creator and providential Sustainer of life. In addition, mankind has been redeemed by God and the Christian entering into this experience believes that his body has become 'the temple of the Holy Spirit'. Thus, Christians 'can claim no inalienable right to death on the grounds that his life is his own, and that after due consideration has been given to the interests of others, he may do with it exactly as he pleases'. Rather 'death signifies the ultimate hopelessness of man before God and his ultimate dependence on God. His faith bids him wait upon God in patience and hope'.[6] It should be borne in mind that, because the Christian believes that man has a future and a destiny in and for God, there can never be complete agreement with those who do not share such beliefs.

Social and Moral Considerations

Society as a whole has an interest in the preservation of life. If the individual's right to die was conceded, it would become necessary to show that society had an overriding interest in the preservation of particular lives and, unless this could be demonstrated, he would be presumed free to exercise his right to die. It would thus be necessary to estimate the value of the individual's life to the community. Even if this were thought morally acceptable, it would cause considerable practical problems. The situation is complicated further by the fact that the phrase 'right to die' is used in a number of different ways. It is used not only to express a demand that a person suffering from an incurable, progressive disease should be free to opt for deliberate death acceleration but also to express a right not to be subjected to inappropriate (death-prolonging) treatment, and the right to receive drugs to control pain even at the risk of shortening life. Such ambiguity emphasizes the complexity of the problem, a fact that needs to be recognized if serious mistakes are not to be made.

Arguments in favour of voluntary euthanasia include progress, compassion, mercy, and that euthanasia is preferable to dying in agony or having useless life artificially prolonged. Arguments based on progress or compassion are, however, spurious, since their practical interpretation depends entirely on whether the concept of voluntary euthanasia is fundamentally acceptable. Only if a 'right to die' is conceded could legislation be considered an advance or its implementation compassionate. Wrongdoing and compassion are mutually exclusive.

Those who argue on grounds of mercy frequently assert that a refusal to countenance voluntary euthanasia demonstrates a callous indifference to suffering. After all, to refuse to put a suffering animal out of its misery would be condemned as cruel. However, unless human beings are regarded merely as animals, it cannot be assumed that what is appropriate treatment for one is necessarily so for the other. The value of human life does not consist simply of a scale of pleasure and pain but in a variety of virtues and graces as well. Furthermore, exposure to suffering is part of the process of maturing, though all would agree that continued meaningless suffering is destructive. Even so, it is a *non sequitur* to conclude that dying patients in persistent pain should be 'put to sleep'.

There is ample evidence to show that pain associated, for example, with advanced cancer may be relieved without resort to an act of deliberate death acceleration.[7] 'The two extremes of dying in pain and being killed do not exhaust the possibilities for the stricken patient'.[8] Even if it were conceded that there may be exceptional cases in which deliberate death acceleration is justified in order to prevent intolerable and uncontrollable suffering, it needs to be asked whether such cases occur in medical practice and whether the ethic of the medical profession can properly regard them as exceptions to the principle of not taking innocent life. There is then the further question whether the law should be altered so as to take account of them. Moreover,

'It is perfectly consistent to argue that morally speaking euthanasia is permissible in some extreme cases, but that it would be wrong to alter the law to allow it in such cases, because this might inescapably, in practice, let in cases in which euthanasia should not be allowed by law. The law is a blunt instrument for dealing with moral complexities and it is better to allow hard cases to be taken care of by the various expedients that are available than to introduce a new principle which would turn out to be too permissive.'[9]

It is sometimes claimed that 'the lethal terminal dose' is already administered under the guise of relieving pain, so that a change in the law would 'tidy up' the present state of affairs and protect the doctor against the possibility of a charge of homicide. It is doubtful whether many, if any, doctors administer narcotic analgesics in such a way as to precipitate death deliberately. On the other hand, to relieve the pain of a dying patient is undoubtedly proper medical treatment, and to term such treatment as 'indirect euthanasia'[10] is both misleading and incorrect. Giving drugs to relieve pain cannot be equated with giving a lethal dose deliberately to end life. Sometimes the use of a narcotic analgesic may marginally shorten the patient's life, but if given for sound medical reasons and in an appropriate dose, the giving of such a drug plays no part in the *legal* causation of death. Nor is the *moral* equivalent of killing the patient deliberately, as the drug is given for the relief of pain. If the patient dies as a result, it is considered from a moral viewpoint to be a secondary effect – foreseeable maybe, but not directly intended.

This 'principle of double effect', although not popular among philosphers because of its potential for abuse, is one with which we have to live in an imperfect world. It applies to all areas of medical and surgical practice. *All* treatment has an inherent risk; a greater risk is acceptable in more extreme situations. It is, however, axiomatic that even in extreme situations the least drastic remedy should be employed. Moreover, correctly used, narcotic analgesics are safer than commonly supposed[11] and there is evidence that those whose pain is relieved may outlive others whose nutrition and rest is disturbed by peristent pain.

Practical Considerations

Requests for 'euthanasia' are made occasionally by patients but experience suggests that they are usually a symptom of unrelieved physical distress or underlying anxiety. Most commonly, it reflects fears about future suffering which may never arise, or need arise, if the patient is properly cared for. Alternatively, the patient may be depressed or just feeling unwanted; he may feel that he is a burden on his relatives or a 'nuisance' to the ward staff. Once the cause of the request has been discovered and dealt with, there is rarely a further request. For those who consistently favour euthanasia, even when they are well cared for, a final demand generally remains something that is for another time – 'not now, of course, later, when things get worse'.

There is, however, a very small minority of elderly patients who appear to have decided that their time has come and that they now wish to die. Although not confused, they seldom express it in words, but make their intention plain by their refusal to eat or drink or co-operate in any treatment.[12] These people are not, however, saying 'Kill me', but simply 'Let me die'. If they become distressed or restless they can be made comfortable, a course of action which leaves them free to change their minds at any time should they wish to, or allows them to die peacefully in their own time.

Arguments Against Legalization

Secondary arguments against voluntary euthanasia may be considered under five headings:

Effects on Patients

The existence of legal euthanasia might undermine the patient's morale and determination by providing 'an easy way out'. This would mean that the patient had less reason for accepting discomfort of any kind, which could in fact increase the pain experienced. Further, the aged and infirm, imagining that they were a burden to their relatives, might feel obliged to ask for euthanasia.

Effects on Doctors and Nurses

Instead of acting only to conserve and to relieve, doctors and nurses would acquire a second role – that of licensed killers. This would certainly jeopardize relationships with many of their patients. Even without legal euthanasia, tablets, elixirs and injections are sometimes refused by those in pain because they fear the possibility of being 'put down'. This would happen more often if voluntary euthanasia were permissible.

Effect on Society

Many questions remain unanswered. Would legalization result in a change of attitude by society towards the life of the individual, towards the elderly and the infirm, towards the terminally ill? If social unrest increases and families continue to disintegrate would there be a growing number of people demanding their 'right to die'? Would the present impetus to improve geriatric and terminal care continue? Would voluntary lead to compulsory, just as therapeutic abortion has in some places led to a policy of abortion on demand? For some, voluntary euthanasia is undoubtedly the thin edge of the wedge. Ultimately the presence of pain or crippling disability would not be necessary; 'uselessness' would suffice. At the inaugural meeting of the British Euthanasia Society, the chairman said:

'Today we are concerned only with voluntary euthanasia; but as public opinion develops, and it becomes possible to form a truer estimate of the value of human life, further progress along preventative lines will be possible. . . . The population is an ageing one, with a larger relative proportion of elderly persons, individuals who have reached a degenerative stage of life. Thus the total amount of suffering and the number of useless lives must increase'.[13]

Similar sentiments were expressed at the first annual general meeting of the American Euthanasia Society.[14]

There are further possible extensions of legalized voluntary euthanasia. For example, suggestions have been made for delayed euthanasia, using anaesthesia with the guarantee of non-arousal, so that useful experiments could be made on human material.[15] Nevertheless, however much the candidate might wish his body to be used in this way, it would undoubtedly cheapen attitudes to human life in general, which would, in turn lead to a less caring and concerned society.

Administrative Problems

Further, if the majority of doctors declined, on conscientious grounds to administer euthanasia, would the State turn to others to execute requests? Current thinking by some of the leading members of the Voluntary Euthanasia Society favours such a course. A request from the patient, either direct or via the family would result in a visit from an inspector from the Euthanasia office of the Department of Health and Social Security. The inspector would assess the situation and, if the established criteria were fulfilled, he would arrange for someone other than the patient's doctor to administer the *coup de grace*.[16] As Sir George Thomson observed: 'To ask a doctor to kill his own patients is too much like asking a sea captain to sink his own ship'.[17] As yet, however, no one has suggested the establishment of special units – Thanatoria – to overcome the practical and emotional problems that might arise if euthanasia were to be administered in the patient's home.

Adequacy of Safeguards

It is generally agreed that if euthanasia were made legal, safeguards to prevent abuse would be necessary. To make euthanasia legal without having considered the practical implications would be folly. Lord Raglan, who introduced the 1969 Bill, has since concluded that it may be an insuperable problem to draw up a suitable declaration; 'All the attempts that I've seen at drawing up a declaration had too many weaknesses for my liking and too many holes picked in them'.[18]

To summarize: to justify, even on pragmatic grounds, a change in the law it would be necessary to show that a change would remove greater evils than it would cause. It is suggested that a careful consideration of the points raised above lead to the conclusion that no such justification exists. 'In the rare cases (if such there are) in which it can be justified morally, it is better for medical men to do all that is necessary to ensure peaceful dying, and to rely on the flexibilities in the administration of the law which even now exist, than to legalize euthanasia (which would have to be subject to rigid formalities and safeguards) for general use'.[19]

Euthanasia is ultimately a policy based on despair, arising from an attitude which implies 'there is nothing more we can do for you'. But Dr. Cicely Saunders, inspired by Christian ideals, has demonstrated at St. Christopher's Hospice, London, that such a statement need never be true; there is always something the good doctor and the good nurse can do.[20, 21] As yet, however, 'intensive preterminal care, although shown to be effective, has barely been explored by society.

The 'Living Will'

Much of the evidence put forward by those in favour of euthanasia, in fact, relates to examples of inappropriate treatment. Fears that they might become victims of 'mindless medicine' have led a number of different groups to produce a document known as a 'living will', the principal clause of which reads,–

'If there is no reasonable prospect of my recovery from physical or mental illness or impairment expected to cause me severe distress or to render me incapable of rational existence, I request that I be allowed to die and not be kept alive by artificial means and that I receive whatever quantity of drugs may be required to keep me free from pain or distress even if the moment of death is hastened'.

Signed: . . . .

The fact that such a step has been considered necessary by a variety of organizations is an indictment of the medical profession. The answer is education not legalization. Generally speaking, it is only in recent years that medical students have received instructions in the art of pain relief. This means that the all too common account of a person dying in agony after weeks or months of unrelieved pain should increasingly be a thing of the past.[22]

Legalization of euthanasia will not correct ignorance about the management of pain and other symptoms or about available supportive resources, nor will it stop mindless medicine. On the other hand, a positive approach to death by society in general together with compassionate, competent medical care and considerate, patient-orientated nursing will do much to overcome the present problems.

Mercy Killing

The killing for merciful motives of a close relative suffering from an irreversible and painful terminal mental or physical disease is treated by English law as murder for which the mandatory sentence is life imprisonment. It has recently been suggested that mercy killing should become a separate criminal offence punishable with a maximum of two years' imprisonment.[23] The Criminal Revision Committee envisages, however, that in practice imprisonment would be imposed in only a few cases. Although the proposal does not seek to legalize mercy killing, there is the danger that such would become its effect in practice. It would not be easy for a jury to distinguish between those to whom the law was really meant to apply and others who might have committed the killing for mixed or even wicked motives. In some cases it would be obvious; in others, however, the line might not be easy to draw and the well-intentioned proposal could open the way for people wanting to get rid of old invalid relatives who had 'outstayed their welcome'. It would add to the fears and anxieties of old people.

Termination of human life – whatever the physical or mental condition of that life – is always a serious matter; its seriousness ought not to be reduced by an amendment of the law which, however well intentioned, could have the effect of making certain kinds of killing seem trivial. It would be better to meet the difficulty which the committee identified by introducing a qualification to the mandatory life sentence for murder, to allow the court discretion in certain cases.[24]

Intensive Care

The Limits of Interference

In 1966 a memorandum on resuscitation after respiratory failure and cardiac arrest was issued by the physician superintendent of Neasden Hospital to all medical officers and senior nursing staff. This stated that:

'The following patients are not to be resuscitated: Very elderly, over 65 years. Malignant disease. Chronic chest disease. Chronic renal failure. Top of yellow treatment card to be marked 'N.T.B.R.' (i.e., not to be resuscitated). The following people should be resuscitated: Collapse as a result of diagnostic or therapeutic procedures – e.g. needle in pleura (even if over 65 years). Sudden unexpected collapse under 65 years – i.e. loss of conscioussness, cessation of breathing, no carotid pulsation'.

The existence of this memorandum was widely discussed by the media and, as a result, the Ministry of Health advised that no patient should be excluded from consideration for resuscitation by reasons of age or diagnostic classification alone, and without regard to all individual circumstances.[25] It is important to note that this is not an instruction recommending indiscriminate or obligatory resuscitation, but rather the reverse. Age or diagnosis alone must not exclude a patient automatically, instead the patient's total situation must be considered including the potential quality of life should he survive. This viewpoint was made clear in a subsequent editorial in *The Lancet*.[26]

Resuscitation is unlikely to succeed where cardiac arrest complicates a progressive downhill course accompanied by serious metabolic disturbances secondary to failing respiration or perfusion. The situation is, of course, different when a fundamental correction can be made in the underlying disturbed physiology, such as correction of hyperkalemia or severe hypokalemia, or the restoration of interrupted ventilation. 'It is part of the clinician's duty to recognize the inevitability of death in certain situations and to avoid the unnecessary physical and emotional trauma associated with unsuccessful attempts at resuscitation in such cases, while at the same time encouraging further effort where some genuine hope is seen to exist'.[27]

The Termination of Artificial Ventilation

If a patient lapses into coma and artificial ventilation is necessary to maintain adequate oxygenation, in what circumstances may the respirator be removed? Ought it to remain until the circulation stops in spite of continued ventilation?

This and other questions raised through the use of respirators were considered in a papal allocution in 1957. The answer given was based on the distinction, already made by Roman Catholic moralists, between 'ordinary' and 'extraordinary' medical procedures. 'Ordinary' is whatever a patient can obtain and undergo without imposing an excessive burden on himself or his family. 'Extraordinary' has been defined as 'Whatever here and now is very costly or very unusual or very painful or very difficult or very dangerous, or if the good effects that can be expected from its use are not proportionate to the difficulty and inconvenience that are entailed.[28] In other words, a doctor has a moral obligation to use ordinary means of preserving life and restoring health but is not bound to institute or persist with extraordinary measures. Apart from the obvious difficulty that the boundary will continue to change as medicine advances and will vary according to national and personal resources, distinguishing between ordinary treatment and treatment that is excessively burdensome is not the best way of resolving the problem. It is more in keeping with clinical realities to regard artificial ventilation as giving the opportunity for a complex attempt at resuscitation. Then, if the patient remains unconscious and incapable of maintaining respiration and circulation without artificial support, it may be said that the attempt at resuscitation has failed; continued ventilation becomes *biologically* inappropriate and the respirator should be removed.

Brain Death

The advent of transplant surgery has complicated decisions about stopping artificial ventilation. For example, surgeons in the United States are no longer willing to transplant a kidney removed after a donor's heart has stopped beating as legal opinion there holds that such an operation would be negligent, in that the chances of success are lower than if the kidney comes from a 'beating-heart' cadaver.[29] Good quality cadaver kidneys are obtainable only in cases where brain death occurs before the heart stops, and the surgeon removes the organs while they are still being oxygenated.

In this situation, the traditional criteria of death – absence of pulse and cessation of respiration – are no longer adequate. Consequently the concept of brain death has been evolved, based on the premise that death of the brain represents death of the individual. During the last decade, as more experience has been acquired, criteria for diagnosing brain death have been clarified. Originally, these included an isoelectric encephalogram for twenty-four hours.[30] Brain death may now, however, be diagnosed without electroencephalography.[31, 32] Other investigations, such as cerebral angiography or cerebral blood flow measurements, are not required.

Recommended clinical criteria varied slightly[31, 32, 33] until the statement by the Conference of British Medical Royal Colleges and their Faculties in 1976.[34] The criteria are designed to confirm whether the patient is in irreversible coma (cortical death) and whether spontaneous respirations and other reflex brain-stem activity has ceased (brain-stem death). Both cortical and brain-stem death must have occurred before a diagnosis of brain death is made. The decision to withdraw artificial support should be made after all the criteria have been fulfilled, and can be made by the consultant in charge (or an experienced deputy) and one other doctor. If transplantation of an organ is involved, neither doctor should be a member of the transplant team.

Although the concept of brain death is not easy to explain to the public, it has been suggested that the example of a guillotine victim might be helpful.[35] Nobody would consider that the decapitated body represented an individual living being; yet the body could be resuscitated and the organs kept alive for a considerable period. Despite such analogies, a gulf will undoubtedly remain for sometime between medical and public concepts of death. Consequently, it may be expected that relatives will be reluctant to consent to the removal of organs from a patient whose heart is still beating. Such reservations must be respected if doctors are to retain people's confidence.

There are rare occasions when irrecoverable brain damage may occur but spontaneous respirations continue. Such cases, in which brain-stem activity is retained, result in an irreversible vegetative state which may last for months. Although there might be no doubt about cortical death it is at present generally agreed that the patient *is* still alive and that it would be unethical to remove organs for transplantation. Instead, the patient should be considered 'terminal' and measures designed to sustain a patient during an acute crisis should not be used.

It should be added that, once the concept of brain death is accepted, there is no fundamental reason why a patient in irreversible coma should not be deemed to have died. In practice, however, the present more stringent criteria for brain death means the likelihood of a mistake being made is considerably reduced. Moreover the practical problems of obtaining the relatives' permission to remove organs for transplantation would be much greater if spontaneous respiration had not ceased.

References

1. *On Dying Well* (1975) *An Anglican Contribution to the Debate on Euthanasia.* London, Church Information Office, p. 51
2. Millard, C. K. (1931) *Euthanasia.* London, C. W. Daniel.
3. Hansard, **368**, 196. *Incurable Patients Bill.* London, HMSO.
4. Nicholson, R. (1975) Should the patient be allowed to die? *Journal of Medical Ethics*, **1**, 5–9.
5. Exodus, **23**, 17; Daniel, **8**, 53.
6. *On Dying Well. Op. cit.*, pp. 16, 19.
7. Saunders, C. M. (1975) The Challenge of Terminal Care in Scientific Foundations of Oncology. (Eds. Symington, T. & Carter, R. L.) London, Heinemann Medical.
8. Horder, Lord Thomas (1936) Speech in House of Lords, December.
9. *On Dying Well. Op. cit.*, p. 12.
10. Fletcher, J. (1970) in *Who Shall Live?* (Ed. Vaux, K.) Philadelphia, Fortress Press.
11. Twycross, R. G. (1975) The use of narcotic analgesics in terminal illness. *Journal of Medical Ethics*, **1**, 14–19.
12. Agate, J. N. (1974) quoted in *On Dying Well*, p. 40.
13. Quoted in St. John-Stevas (1961) *Life, Death and the Law*. London, Eyre and Spottiswoode.
14. New York Times, 27.1.1939.
15. Vere, D. W. (1971) *Should Christians Support Voluntary Euthanasia?* London, C.M.F. Publications.
16. Saul, C. (1976) in Debate on Euthanasia, University Debating Society. February 1976.
17. Thomson, G. (1972) The Euthanasia Debate. *Contact*, **40**, 10–16.
18. Raglan, Lord (1972) The case for voluntary euthanasia in The problem of euthanasia. *Contact*, **39**, 3–11.
19. *On Dying Well. Op. cit.*, p. 62.
20. Saunders, C. M. (1975) *Op. cit.*
21. Lamerton, R. (1973) *Care of the Dying.* London, Priory Press.
22. Twycross, R. G. (1975) Relief of Terminal Pain. *British Medical Journal*, **4**, 212–214.
23. Criminal Law Revision Committee (1976) *Working paper on the offences against the Person*. London, HMSO.
24. Editorial (1976) Too Merciful to Mercy Killers. *The Times*, 29th September.
25. Editorial (1971) Termination of life. *British Medical Journal*, **3**, 187.
26. Editorial (1970) Not strive officiously. *Lancet*, **2**, 915.
27. Editorial (1972) Limitations of Resuscitation. *Lancet*, **1**, 1169–1170.
28. Healey, E. F. (1956) *Medical Ethics.* Loyola University Press.
29. Editorial (1975) Brain Death. *British Medical Journal*, **1**, 356.
30. Harvard Medical School (1968) *Journal of the American Medical Association*, **205**, 340.
31. Editorial (1974) Brain damage and Brain Death. *Lancet*, **1**, 341–342.
32. Editorial (1975) *British Medical Journal*, **1**, 356.
33. Bliss, B. P. & Johnson, A. G. (1975) *Aims and Motives in Clinical Medicine.* London, Pitman Medical.
34. Diagnosis of Brain Death (1976) *British Medical Journal*, **2**, 1187–1188.

35. British Transplant Society (1975) The shortage of organs for clinical transplantation: document for discussion. *British Medical Journal*, 1, 251–256.

Further Reading

Bliss, B. P. & Johnson, A. G. (1975) *Aims and Motives in Clinical Medicine*. London, Pitman Medical.
Downing, A. B. (Ed.) (1969) *Euthanasia and the Right to Death – the case for Voluntary Euthanasia*. London, Peter Owen.
On Dying Well. (1975) An Anglican Contribution to the debate on Euthanasia. London, Church Information Office.
Saunders, C. M. (Ed.) (1978) *The Management of Terminal Disease*. London, Arnold.
Trowell, H. (1973) *The Unfinished Debate on Euthanasia*. London, S.C.M. Press.
Vere, D. W. (1971) *Voluntary Euthanasia – is there an alternative?* London, Christian Medical Fellowship.

8

The Use and Misuse of Drugs
Allister Vale

A drug has been defined as 'any substance or product that is used or intended to be used to modify or explore physiological systems or pathological states for the benefit of the recipient'.[1]

The purpose of using a drug is to bring benefit to the patient but it may also cause harm. Prescribing, therefore, needs to be constantly reviewed. From the ancient past this principle has been recognized and Hippocrates crystallized it in his simple phrases – 'I will maintain the utmost respect for human life' and 'The health of the patient will be my first consideration'.

Conventional medical treatment has three aims – first, the correction of abnormalities; second, the relief of symptoms which they cause; third, the relief of anxiety or mental distress caused by a disease. Whether one or more of these purposes is followed, it should be done only in the patient's interest. It must not be done in the interests of the doctor or any other person, unless the patient agrees to this knowingly and freely.

Before treating any patient with a drug the doctor should have considered the following:[2, 3]

(i) Should he interfere with the patient at all? Does the condition require active intervention? Sometimes it does not: the disability may be self-limiting, available treatment may be inadequate or toxic, or the patient may be unsuitable for physical or psychological reasons.

(ii) If he intervenes what exactly does he hope to achieve?

(iii) Is the drug he has in mind capable of bringing this about and if so, how should it be prescribed to obtain the required result? What evidence of efficacy should be used?

(iv) Is the agent the drug of choice? Are its effects modified by the patient's illness or concurrent medication? Is ancillary medication indicated?

(v) What other effects may the drug have? May they be harmful?

(vi) Does the likelihood of benefit outweigh the likelihood of harm?

In order to ensure the rational use of drugs the doctor must have knowledge of the preparation he intends to prescribe. The growing availability of information in the field of pharmacokinetics,* the type and frequency of drug interactions and adverse effects, and the consequence of variation in the bioavailability** of drugs are factors

* The study of the absorption, distribution, metabolism and excretion of drugs.
** The percentage of drug released from a formulation that becomes available for biological effect.

which all practitioners should take into account when prescribing drugs.

The Drug Explosion

The cost of running the National Health Service has risen annually since its inception in 1948. Expenditure on health and personal social services in England alone is now in excess of £4000 million. Although the proportion spent on the pharmaceutical services has remained at around 10%, the number of prescriptions dispensed by chemists in England has risen considerably; for example, in 1975 there were 282 million prescriptions, an increase of 18 million over the number dispensed in 1969. This means that there are about six prescriptions per year per head of population. Each prescription on average costs the British tax payer £1.30.

It must be remembered, however, that self-medication is even more common than prescribed medication.[4,5,6] In one study for every prescribed item ingested there were two non-prescribed items.[5] These same workers also showed that 80% of adults and 55% of children had taken at least one kind of medicine during the two week study period; more than half of the adults and almost one third of the children had taken medicine within the 24 hours prior to questioning.

There is little doubt that there has been an increase both in the ingestion of prescribed and non-prescribed medication in recent years. There are several reasons for this:

(i) A large number of therapeutically useful preparations have made their appearance during this period.

(ii) An increased life expectancy has produced a change in disease patterns and a rise in the incidence of chronic and degenerative diseases. For example, between 1967 and 1971 there was a 50% and 30% increase respectively in the number of prescriptions for diuretics and preparations used to treat rheumatic disease.

(iii) Although there has been an increase in the number of prescriptions, there is no evidence of an increase in the number of consultations with general practitioners.[7] In other words, an increasing proportion of general practitioner consultations result in a prescription. This suggests that people's expectation about health may be rising and may mean that they are more likely, for example, to regard a headache, as something wrong and seek remedies for symptoms which were formerly accepted as a part of everyday life.

(iv) Between 1961 and 1974 the number of prescriptions for tranquillizers (benzodiazepines, phenothiazines and meprobamate) more than doubled. This trend is discussed below.

The flood of new drugs in recent years has provided many dramatic improvements in therapy but it has also created a number of problems of equal magnitude. As a result the therapeutic revolution has imposed on doctors a compelling responsibility to use drugs wisely.

Legislative Control of Drugs

Patients in Great Britain are rightly protected from many of the dangers of self-medication in that the majority of potentially toxic substances are available only on prescription. The sale or supply of medicines is controlled by Part III of the Medicines Act 1968 and by orders made under it. The basic principle is that a medicinal product may only be sold from a registered pharmacy under the supervision of a pharmacist, unless it is on a General Sale List, or is subject to some other exemption under the Act. There are three classes of product under the Medicines Act 1968 namely, General Sale List Medicines, Pharmacy Medicines and Prescription Only Medicines.

While the Medicines Act 1968 is concerned with regulating the legitimate use of medicinal products, the primary purpose of the Misuse of Drugs Act 1971 is to prevent the abuse of 'controlled drugs'. Under this Act a doctor, dentist or veterinary surgeon acting in his professional capacity is able to prescribe, administer, manufacture or supply a controlled drug (Schedules 2 and 3, Misuse of Drugs Regulations, 1973).

The Regulations made under the 1971 Act – The Misuse of Drugs Regulations 1973 – lists drugs under four schedules. Schedule 1 contains preparations which can be bought, sold or possessed without prescription whereas Schedules, 2 and 3 contain drugs which can only be prescribed by a registered practitioner. Schedule 2 includes the opiates and major stimulant drugs such as amphetamine; Schedule 3 includes benzphetamine and mephentermine; Schedule 4 contains hallucinogenic drugs such as LSD and cannabis.

The Misuse of Drugs (Notification of a supply to Addicts) Regulations 1973 make it obligatory for a doctor to furnish details to the Chief Medical Officer at the Home Office of any person whom he considers, or has reasonable grounds to suspect, to be addicted to any 'controlled' drug listed in the Schedule to these Regulations (this includes all opiates, cocaine and methadone). Under these regulations it is an offence for a doctor to prescribe heroin or cocaine and their derivatives for the satisfaction of an addiction other than under a licence issued by the Secretary of State.

Information on Drugs

Becker *et al.*[8] have shown that prescribing patterns are determined by educational experience. It is therefore significant that about 70% of all currently marketed drugs were unknown or unavailable when more than half of the doctors prescribing today were receiving, or had already completed, their medical training.[9] Where, then, do doctors obtain information about new drugs?

The pharmaceutical industry remains a most important source, especially for general practitioners. Mailings of drug notices and advertisements are numerous and the majority of professional journals carry advertisements of pharmaceutical products. In addition, there are many journals and newspapers with a controlled circulation which are sent free to doctors and supported entirely by drug advertising. Unfortunately, many advertisements give insufficient information to help the practitioner make a decision on prescribing.[10]

The Association of the British Pharmaceutical Industry (ABPI) has recently made available an Annual Compendium of the data sheets on a large proportion of proprietary drugs, which contains more information than is available in MIMS (Monthly Index of Medical Specialities). In 1968 the ABPI established a Medical-Pharmaceutical Forum and it also supports the Office of Health Economics (OHE) which publishes papers on health problems. Pharmaceutical companies also organize or sponsor postgraduate meetings at national and regional levels which provide much useful information on new advances in therapy. The medical representative, however, remains the cornerstone and probably the most effective means (as far as his employers are concerned) of disseminating information on a company's products. Occasionally, a representative will invite a doctor (and sometimes his spouse) to join him for lunch or dinner 'to discuss this further'. If such invitations are accepted, practitioners need to be on their guard against agreeing, at the end of the meal, to 'give the drug a try' unless an outstanding pharmacological case has been made for its use.

Despite the contribution which the pharmaceutical industry is making in this sphere, it is obviously preferable that doctors should learn the virtues of new drugs from less biased sources. It is therefore to be regretted that so few alternative sources of effective information on new drugs are in fact available (one notable exception is the Drug and Therapeutics Bulletin published by the Consumers Association). The Department of Health and Social Security (DHSS) sponsors the Prescribers Journal but this contains reviews of aspects of therapeutics rather than information on new drugs. Hospital based, regionally co-ordinated Drug Information Services are now being established throughout Great Britain and should provide valuable unbiased information on drugs.

At a more personal level it has been shown that a powerful influence on prescribing patterns in general practice is the advice given by hospital consultants.[11] It is therefore important that the therapeutic needs of patients are very carefully assessed before their discharge from hospital.

It should be the desire of every doctor to keep abreast of developments in therapeutics so that he may give his patients the best and most appropriate treatment. Consequently, there will be a strong motivation to read the journals and to attend postgraduate meetings.

Appropriate Use of Drugs

Choice of Treatment

Planning a course of treatment involves not only the selection of the most suitable medicine, but also the dosage form, dose frequency, duration and, not least, a decision on when and how the course should end. A doctor should prescribe well-tried remedies with which he is familiar and avoid using newer ones unless there is good evidence of a significant advantage. Only then should a new drug be incorporated into his therapeutic armoury. The serious side effects of new drugs may not be apparent until several years after their release (for example, the side effects of the β-blocker, practolol). As most new drugs lack major advantages,[12] the enthusiasm with which many are received is often misplaced. In general, there is little to be gained from substituting a new drug for another of the same group when the latter has failed to produce a response. When once established a treatment regime should not be changed without very good reasons.

In recent years several pharmaceutical companies have invited general practitioners to assist in the evaluation of new drugs and in return have given them a fee, a gift or an invitation to attend a conference abroad. Not only may the scientific quality of many of these trials be questioned but it is known also that for an investment of perhaps £100,000 a company might hope to create a £1 million annual market. This occurs for two reasons. First, doctors may be persuaded to use the drug when the results of the trial are published in a (usually commercially sponsored) medical journal; secondly, as many as 60% of patients given a new treatment in one of these trials remain on the drug thereafter.

The main objection to such trials is that in many cases the choice of treatment is dictated not by what is best for the patient but either by what the pharmaceutical company desires or, at worst, by the prospect of financial gain. Furthermore, it is clearly unethical for a patient whose symptoms are well controlled on one drug to be changed to another, which may have no therapeutic advantages or even produce greater side effects, without his consent being obtained, which it often is not.

It is imperative that a doctor should carefully consider the choice of treatment. He should not be swayed by every wind of therapeutic change or by the pharmaceutical companies unless a new drug has been shown to have distinct advantages.

Non-compliance with prescribing instructions is a common cause of undertreatment or treatment failure. Out-patient experience suggests that as many as 50% of patients do not take the prescribed treatment, or do not follow the suggested dosage regime. On each occasion, therefore, that a prescription is written the drug regime should be reviewed. This is particularly important in elderly patients who may experience toxic side-effects at 'normal' dose levels. Predisposing factors which may lead to non-compliance include unpleasant medication, complicated dosage schedules, multiple drug regimes and awareness of side effects. Hence simple regimens and warnings of anticipated side-effects which often wear off may lead to greater patient compliance.

Before commencing treatment it is always wise to ask how the results will be evaluated? Whenever possible some measurement of the severity of the disease, however simple, should be obtained. It may be for example, the measurement of the haemoglobin concentration in iron deficiency anaemia; of grip strength in rheumatoid arthritis; or the size of a secondary neoplasm or mass of glands when cytotoxic therapy is to be given. Alternatively a chart may be kept by the patient of the frequency of attacks of migraine, angina or fits. Adjustments in the dosage of medication can then be made on the basis of this objective evidence.

Adverse Effects

Dunlop[13] has suggested that 'perhaps some five per cent of the beds in our general hospitals are occupied by patients suffering to a greater or lesser extent from our attempts to treat them'. In the USA the Food and Drug Administration has estimated that one in seven of all hospital beds in that country are occupied by patients under treatment for adverse reactions caused by drugs.[14] Melmon[15] has calculated that the economic losses due to adverse drug reactions in the United States now amount to 3000 million dollars each year.

All treatments carry some risk, but many unwanted effects of drugs can be predicted from their pharmacological action and hence avoided. Regrettably, many doctors are unfamiliar with these basic principles. Some patients are treated with several drugs at the same time, either to minimize the side effects of one drug, to produce an effect which is unavailable from a single agent, or because a patient has several diseases each of which requires treatment. Drug interactions have therefore become an important problem. Various books and a number of Drug Discs have recently been produced which provide a ready source of information on such interactions.

It is imperative from the point of view of the safety and welfare of our patients and the economic cost involved that everything in our power is done to reduce the incidence and severity of adverse drug reactions. Vere[16] has suggested ways in which this might be done.

Inappropriate Treatment

Some treatments are inappropriate. It is not, for example, uncommon for a patient with a 'cold' or sore throat to visit his general practitioner and ask for an antibiotic. The fact that in 1974, 38 million prescriptions for antibiotics were dispensed indicates that he is as likely as not to come away with a prescription for such a drug. (In some parts of Europe, chloramphenicol is commonly prescribed for 'influenza-like' illnesses, a practice which is clearly indefensible.) The disappearance of symptoms within three or four days is then attributed by the patient to the wonders of modern medicine rather than to the natural remission of their disease.

In recent years the hazards of barbiturates have been increasingly recognized in misuse by young people, the dependence of the middle-aged and elderly and ingestion by parasuicidal and suicidal patients. These hazards – and the fact that safer alternatives are available – prompted the establishment of the Campaign on the Use and Restriction of Barbiturates (CURB) which succeeded in some measure in obtaining a voluntary ban on the prescribing of barbiturates as sedatives, hypnotics and anxiolytic agents. The main difficulty in achieving a total ban on the use of these drugs except in epilepsy and anaesthesia is to persuade patients who have become dependent upon barbiturates to change to a safer alternative.

It has sometimes been claimed that succumbing to pressure from the patient or his relatives for treatment is, in effect, therapeutic. The patient's need is fulfilled or his relatives beliefs are satisfied. This is therefore regarded as acceptable, if not necessarily the best medicine. The moral principle which condemns inappropriate treatment is enshrined in the Declaration of Geneva which states 'the health of my patients will be my first consideration'. The health of my patient can never extend to succumbing to his unwise or irrational demands for treatment. Patient pressure (and the inducement of financial gain) must be subordinated to the *real* needs of our patients.

A further aspect of inappropriate treatement is overprescribing. Dunlop[17] believes that, 'we do not always draw a clear distinction between the patient's 'wants' and what we think are his 'needs' and it is regrettable how much we accede to the patient's demands in order to placate him and to save ourselves time and trouble. The virtual elimination of the financial barrier between the physician and the patient, the result of the National Health Service, in which the manufacturer produces, the doctor orders, the patient consumes and the government pays, though salutory in many respects, has also encouraged overprescribing'.

Thomson[18] has suggested that before a prescription is written the following guidelines should be borne in mind: (1) Is it really necessary? (2) Never prescribe more than is absolutely necessary (3)

Always prescribe the cheapest effective drug by its approved name. (4) Never indulge in polypharmacy if it can possibly be avoided.

Withdrawal of Treatment

Elaborate and unnecessary drug regimes can and should be withdrawn when progressive deterioration, often with multiple organ failure, sets in. It is sometimes said that withdrawing 'treatment' removes the patient's hope. This need not be the case if the distinction between 'treatment' and 'care' is realized. Care consists of symptomatic relief, skilled nursing and nutrition. This, in contrast to unnecessary drug therapy, should never be withdrawn.

Cost-benefit Analysis (see p. 153)

Before a drug or treatment is chosen a profit and loss account (cost-benefit analysis) should be drawn up on the patient's behalf. Some doctors appear to have an innate ability to assess the integrated effect of the benefits and risks of therapeutic procedure when they decide either to treat or to withhold treatment. Too often, however, judgements of this type are made without detailed analysis of all the relevant factors, which should include the likely benefits, the risks, the costs and the patient's social and mental resources. In recent years methods of dealing with such complex therapeutic decisions in an explicit and logical fashion have been developed (see, for example, Pauker and Kassirer[19]).

In summary, 'treatment failures are often due to lack of compliance, errors in diagnosis, and inadequate adjustment of dosage. Careful prescribing can improve the results of treatment and reduce the incidence of adverse reactions to drugs; in addition, if close attention is paid to limiting the duration of treatment and the relative cost of drugs of the same class, a lot of money can be saved'.[20]

Misuse of Drugs

As Dunnell and Cartwright[21] have shown, medicine-taking is a common activity, frequently indulged in, often for long periods. It serves a variety of needs, many of them social and psychological rather than purely therapeutic.

Psychotropic Agents

The use of these agents and particularly of the benzodiazepine groups of drugs (e.g. diazepam, chlordiazepoxide, nitrazepam) is increasing. As Wade[22] has suggested there are two features of their use which are a warning that misuse is occurring:
(i) A high proportion of patients once started on these drugs cannot

be weaned off them, although there is no conventional evidence of addiction such as a desire to increase the dose or liability to suffer withdrawal symptoms.

(ii) An increasing proportion of the population enjoying good physical health is demanding these drugs.

Why are psychotropic drugs so frequently prescribed?

It has been suggested that both the medical profession and society are exposed to the influences of the pharmaceutical companies who appear to be 'redefining and labelling as medical problems a wide range of human behaviour which, in the past, has been viewed as falling within the bounds of normal trials and tribulations of human existence'.[23]

This, however, is a dangerous view. Lennard believes that when a physician 'prescribes a drug for the control or solution or both of personal problems of living he does more than merely relieve the discomfort caused by the problem. He simultaneously communicates a model for an acceptable and useful way of dealing with personal and interpersonal problems'. As a result many patients now expect their doctors to prescribe psychotropic agents for problems which are insoluble by drug therapy. It is because of a lack of time and the facility or desire to provide other alternatives that many practitioners succumb to their patient's expectations. Franz Kafka made his country doctor say: 'To write prescriptions is easy but to come to an understanding with people is hard'. Doctors may therefore be inadvertently encouraging the misuse of drugs because it is easier to prescribe them than to discuss a patient's problems.

What then should a practitioner's attitude be to the use of psychotropic agents? Vere[24] offers a good summary, 'A doctor will want in general to offer treatment only when he has a precise diagnosis. . . . He will want the diagnosis to comprise physical, mental and spiritual aspects. He can then direct his drugs, if they are needed, like bullets towards defined targets. These targets will be: (a) to restore towards normality, for that person, physical and mental function so as (b) to permit, but not influence, the emergence and relief of his spiritual problems. This is where the supernatural aspect enters, not in the medicine itself, which has a permissive or adjuvant role, but because there was no hope of clearing up spiritual difficulties as long as body and mind could not function to allow them to be expressed. These are therapeutic aims, in the proper sense of that word . . . so our aims should not comprise the contemporarily acceptable non-therapeutic aims, or patients' aberrant requests – to provide pleasure, an experience, a thrill, an escape from difficulties, or a means of self-punishment or self-justification or a means to modify one's personality. The aim is to subdue mental disorder so that a man's real self, and its spiritual problems, can emerge. The goal and extent of therapy will be limited by the revealed nature of man's life. Maybe the chosen drug will, in the end, be the same but the reasons for giving it and the follow-up on its effects will differ. The prescriber will wish to avoid treatments which cultivate false attitudes to life, such as those which help to evade problems, or make work absence seem respectable, or assist suicide, or boost sales on a black market'.

The story of man's resort to pharmacologically active substances stretches back into the earliest history. 'Human kind,' wrote T. S. Eliot, 'cannot bear very much reality'. Unfortunately, psychotropic medicines are being increasingly used as a palliative for the treatment of man's inability to come to terms with his environment and himself.

Parasuicide

In 1975 more than 100,000 patients were admitted to hospitals in England and Wales as a result of an acute poisoning episode. The majority of these were not attempting suicide but were indulging in a conscious, impulsive, manipulative act undertaken to secure redress of an intolerable situation which, for the particular individual in question, cannot be or has not been relieved by more rational means. Kreitman *et al*.[25] have proposed the term parasuicide to describe what has now become almost an acceptable form of social behaviour. There are two main motives. First, an attempt to obtain relief or the interruption of a stressful situation; second, the desire for attention after more conventional means of securing it have failed – the 'cry for help'. In almost every case parasuicidal patients ingest therapeutic preparations: those between 15 and 35 years predominantly take psychotropic agents, whereas older patients ingest barbiturates and non-barbiturate hypnotics.[26]

Prescribing habits and the overprescription of drugs and, as a result, their hoarding, either wilfully or thoughtlessly, are factors in determining the means of parasuicide. However, the main reason for the dramatic increase in the number of parasuicides is probably the breakdown in family life and of the family itself as the basic unit of society. Family disintegration, unsatisfactory marital relationships, and 'adolescent turmoil' are often the background of parasuicidal patients. The concepts which gave strength and stability to society in the past were largely inculcated in the home. The strong ties which kept families together ensured that when 'adolescent turmoil' arose (as indeed it must), someone was at hand to respond to the 'cry for help'.

Drug Dependence

Drug dependence has been defined as a 'state, psychic and sometimes also physical, resulting in the interaction between a living organism and a drug, characterized by behaviour and other responses which will always include a compulsion to take the drug on a continuous or periodic basis in order to experience its psychic effects and sometimes to avoid the discomfort of its absence. Tolerance may or may not be present'.[27]

Drug dependence is not a new phenomenon but the abuse of drugs, has, at least in Great Britain been uncommon until recent years. Before World War II, addiction to opiates was largely confined to those who had acquired their drug habit in the course of treatment for various painful illnesses, and those whose professional work brought them into contact with dangerous drugs and to whom the drugs were therefore readily available in times of personal crisis.

Throughout the 1950s opiate drug abusers known to the Home Office were predominantly individuals of a literary and artistic background. In the years that followed, however, opiate dependence spread throughout the social classes and in 1976 1881 addicts were known to the Home Office to be receiving narcotic drugs; the majority of these addicts were between 25 and 28 years of age.

In contrast to the relatively small number of opiate addicts a BBC (Midweek) Survey[28] has suggested that 'soft' drug use is very prevalent in society. The survey deduced evidence that 3.8 million people in the United Kingdom had used cannabis, 657,000 had used LSD, just under 1.3 million had used amphetamines and 582,000 had used hypnotics – both the last two drugs without prescription. Bewley[29] has estimated that 50–100 per 100,000 population are dependent on amphetamines, 1000–2000 per 100,000 population are dependent on barbiturates, and 50–150 per 100,000 population are regular users of cannabis.

The widespread use of 'soft' drugs raises the question of whether or not such mind-altering agents should be freely available. Fundamentally, this is the matter of the freedom of the individual to do what he wants. In our society at present freedom is rightly constrained in many ways both to protect the individual from unacceptable risk (e.g. heroin abuse) and to benefit the community (e.g. payment of taxes). Society, through the various agencies to which it delegates responsibility, decides the constraints on this freedom and imposes them by legislation. Some would argue that because many thousands smoke 'pot' in spite of current legislation, the law should be relaxed. This does not, however, follow. Mass law breaking (e.g. petty thieving, exceeding the speed limit and tax evasion) is in itself no good reason for changing the law. If 'pot' smoking was completely harmless to the individual and society then the law would be unjust and unreasonable. It is likely, however, that any drug capable of producing a pleasurable state of mind would be subject to considerable use, and therefore abuse, with resulting psychological and physical effects. Society has to decide whether the individual and collective benefits outweigh the risk. Many believe they do not.

Boyd[30] considers that very few of those addicted to drugs, particularly opiates, can be considered either psychotic or psychopathic. He believes there is, 'a profound social isolation in which, even within their own subculture, self-concern, self-determination and personal hedonism massively prevail. Yet close to the surface there is tremendous guilt accompanied by intense self-criticism and awareness of emptiness, ineffectiveness and failure'.

Vere[31] has suggested four possible factors in the aetiology of drug dependence.

(i) A search for a 'prop' upon which to depend. Many believe that the centre of the 'drug problem' is the drug. Yet more often it is the drug-taker who is most of the problem, and was so before he ever took the drug. It is true that some drugs are strongly addictive. But it is also true that most of those who are now 'hooked' on them were deliberately seeking this. It is interesting to note that opiates taken for severe pain seldom lead to dependence or to pleasure in those who need them. Yet as a rule, opiates taken for their other actions evoke dependence. Clearly it is not the drug alone which is to blame.

(ii) A desire to modify the mind. This may be to avoid misery or to gain a transcendental experience. For others it may merely be escape from the boredom of their motiveless living.[32]

(iii) A desire to compensate for real or imagined rejection.

(iv) A desire to 'resocialize' – to identify with a group. This is the obverse of (iii). Drug-dependents often describe this as a chief reason for choosing drugs. Their desire is to belong to a group with a common language and interest.

The view is often expressed today that there is little wrong in being 'hooked' by a habit, pleasure or drug so long as no one else gets harmed. 'What is wrong, the argument goes, with being dependent if as a result life is more satisfying than it would otherwise have been? It is up to each person what he does; he knows what suits him best'.

There are two objections to this view. First, most people would agree that distorted dependence damages. 'It can narrow the personality, shutting it up to a mere habit which pre-empts attention, resources, learning and emotional life. It can enslave. It can often destroy people mentally and physically. The alcoholic with liver disease and the smoker with lung cancer . . . are examples of those who have not lived to the full. . . . True, some forms of dependence are less costly. Take, for example, the large numbers of unhappy, middle-aged women who take sleeping pills and tranquillizers too frequently. But even that is an enormous expense to them or the NHS and involves their doctors in a morass of unnecessary medication.[33]

The second objection stems from the Christian belief that because God is the Author and Giver of Life, it is wrong for man to spoil or destroy it without a divine mandate. On this view a man is not his own, to please himself about what he may do with his body, his mind or his possessions, Seen in this light the problem of distorted dependence takes on a new and obviously spiritual dimension.

References

1. WHO (1966) WHO scientific group on principles for pre-clinical testing of drug safety. *W.H.O. Technical Report Series*, 341, 7.
2. Laurence, D. R. (1975) in *Advanced Medicine: Topics in Therapeutics*, 1, 138. Tunbridge Wells, Pitman Medical.
3. Binns, T. B. (1975) Sensible prescribing. *Practitioner*, 214, 118.
4. Jefferys, M., Brotherston, J. H. F. & Cartwright, A. (1969) Consumption of medicines on a working-class housing estate. *British Journal of Preventive and Social Medicine*, 14, 64.
5. Wadsworth, M. E. J., Butterfield, W. J. H. & Blaney, R. (1971) *Health and Sickness: The Choice of Treatment*. London, Tavistock.
6. Dunnell, K. & Cartwright, A. (1972) *Medicine Takers, Prescribers and Hoarders*. London, Routledge and Kegan Paul.
7. R.C.G.P. (1970) *Present State and Future Needs in General Practice*. Reports from General Practice, No. 13, 2nd Edn. London, R.C.G.P.
8. Becker, M. H., Stolley, P. D., Lasagna, L., McEvilla, J. D. & Sloane, L. M. (1972) Differential education concerning therapeutics and resultant physician prescribing patterns. *Journal of Medical Education*, 47, 118.
9. Parish, P. A. (1971) The prescribing of psychotropic drugs in general practice. *Journal of the Royal College of General Practitioners*, 21, Supplement 4, 60.
10. Stimson, G. V. (1975) Information contained in drug advertisements. *British Medical Journal*, 4, 508.
11. Becker, *et al.*, *Op. cit.*
12. NEDO (1973) *Innovative Activity in the Pharmaceutical Industry*. London, HMSO.
13. Dunlop, D. (1969) Adverse effects of drugs. *British Medical Journal*, 2, 622.
14. U.S. Dept. of Health, Education and Welfare (1969) *Task Force on Prescription Drugs: Final Report*. Washington, D.C.
15. Melmon, K. L. (1971) Preventable drug reactions – causes and cures. *New England Journal of Medicine*, 284, 1361.
16. Vere, D. W. (1976) Risks of everyday life – drugs. *Proceedings of the Royal Society of Medicine*, 69, 106.
17. Dunlop, D. (1970) Abuse of drugs by the public and doctors. *British Medical Bulletin*, 26, 236.
18. Thomson, W. A. R. (1977) *A Dictionary of Medical Ethics and Practice*. Bristol, John Wright.
19. Pauker, S. G. & Kassirer, J. P. (1975) Therapeutic decision making: a cost-benefit analysis. *New England Journal of Medicine*, 293, 229.
20. Editorial (1976) Care in prescribing. *British Medical Journal*, 1, 413.
21. Dunnell, K. & Cartwright, A. (1972) *Op. cit.*
22. Wade, O. L. (1973) in The medical use of psychotropic drugs. *Journal of the Royal College of General Practitioners*, 23, Supplement 2, 65.
23. Lennard, H. L., Epstein, L. J., Bernstein, A. & Ransom, D. C. (1971) *Mystification and Drug Misuse*. San Francisco, Jossey-Bass.
24. Vere, D. W. (1971) Psychopharmacology and moral responsibility. *In the Service of Medicine*, 67, 8.

25. Kreitman, N., Philip, A. E., Greer, S. & Bagley, C. R. (1969) Parasuicide. *British Journal of Psychiatry*, **115**, 746.
26. Vale, J. A. (1977) The epidemiology of acute poisoning. *Acta Pharmacologica et Toxicologica,* **41**, Supplement 2, 443.
27. WHO (1969) Report of expert committee on addiction-producing drugs. *Technical Report Series*, **341**, 7. Geneva, WHO.
28. BBC (Midweek) Survey (1973) London, The Social Research Design Consultancy.
29. Bewley, T. H. (1972) Personal communication quoted in Willis, J. H. *Drug Dependence*. London, Faber.
30. Boyd, P. (1975) Problems and treatment of drug abuse in adolescence. *Proceedings of the Royal Society of Medicine*, **68**, 566.
31. Vere, D. W. (1975) in *The Abuse of Drugs* (Eds. Potts, D. & Vere, D. W.). London, Intervarsity Press.
32 Nicholi, A. (1972) Paper given at the Fourth International Congress of Christian Physicians, Toronto, Canada.
33. Vere, D. W. (1975) *Op. cit.*

9

Problems in Clinical Psychiatry
David Toms

In psychiatry, which is a relatively new and growing discipline, there are a number of recurring ethical issues. Psychiatry has its roots in Medicine and the model of the doctor-patient relationship still strongly affects its practice. The main difference is the degree of trust and dependence the patient puts in the doctor and his treatment. In medicine the patient sees his problem objectively and 'hands over' both himself and it to the doctor for treatment. In psychiatry, however, treatment necessarily includes the concepts of personal freedom and growth, and demands an active personal participation by the patient.

Hospital Admission

Another important difference arises from the physician's statutory responsibilities under the Mental Health Act (1959).[1] Until reform commenced one hundred years ago mentally ill people were restrained and locked up in large custodial institutions outside the large towns. Those who cared for them were called 'alienists'. Even today 5–10% of the most disturbed psychiatric patients are admitted to hospital compulsorily to start their treatment. In most cases Sections 29 and 30 of the Act, (retaining a patient in an emergency for three days) or the observation order Section 25 for twenty-eight days allow sufficient progress for a therapeutic relationship to be established.

When liberty is restored the patient usually continues treatment. In severe psychiatric disorders where insight is lacking and the disturbance is recurrent and/or longstanding, the Section 26 order can impose continued compulsory treatment for one year. During this time rehabilitation may proceed to outpatient supervision under the control of the Responsible Medical Officer (RMO). This order requires agreement of the next of kin and/or a Social Worker and, in addition, two medical recommendations, one of which must be from a doctor who is recognized as being specially experienced. This is usually the psychiatrist in charge (RMO). The second recommendation is signed preferably by the patient's general practitioner. This detention can be terminated by the RMO whenever he is satisfied that the patient has recovered and will continue to co-operate with any essential treatment. The RMO will normally respond with sympathy to a request from the next of kin who wishes to take responsibility for the patient again and there is an appeal arrangement to an independent Mental Health Review Tribunal.

When mentally ill people are brought before the Crown Court or a higher Court for offences due to, or affected by, their illness the Court may impose a Section 60 order for one year's treatment if recommended by the reporting psychiatrist. This functions almost identically with a Section 26 order and the RMO can again discharge the patient whenever he is well. Violent and dangerous mentally ill offenders may be detained under Her Majesty's pleasure under the control of the Home Secretary using Section 65 of the Mental Health Act (1959).

The Patient's Liberty

The ethical issue here is the removal of personal liberty because a psychiatrist has diagnosed mental illness, subnormality or a psychopathic disorder (in a patient under 21 years of age) likely to respond to treatment. Gostin,[2] a lawyer for the National Association of Mental Health (NAMH) in this country and Szasz[3] in America, question this power which society gives to psychiatrists. Most doctors would exercize this power of compulsory restraint with caution and then only on a person who was ill and whose illness placed his life, or the lives of those around him, in danger. They would also wish to predict whether such a patient would be likely to respond to treatment and thereby be restored to his former life and family but they would avoid becoming involved in family quarrels or sectarian interests or where there is no convincing evidence that mental illness is present.

With regard to the question of the patient's personal freedom it is important to remember that he must give permission for any procedure or treatment unless he lacks the capacity to express his own wishes or is a severe threat to others, and secondly, that the patient must be released as soon as the conditions for compulsory treatment no longer apply.

A clear statement of the position was made by the World Psychiatric Association in the *Declaration of Hawaii 1977* (see p. 197), the preamble of which is reproduced here and I believe it should be fully supported.

'Ever since the dawn of culture, ethics has been an essential part of the healing art. Conflicting loyalties for physicians in contemporary society, the delicate nature of the therapist-patient relationship, and the possibility of abuses of psychiatric concepts, knowledge and technology in actions contrary to the laws of humanity, all make high ethical standards more necessary than ever for those practising the art and science of psychiatry.

As a practitioner of medicine and a member of society the psychiatrist has to consider the ethical demands on all physicians and the societal duties of every man and woman. A keen conscience and personal judgment is essential for ethical behaviour. Nevertheless, to clarify the profession's ethical implications and to guide individual psychiatrists and help form their consciences, written rules are needed'.

Some special points in the Declaration are worth emphasizing:

1. The aim of psychiatry is to promote personal growth towards mature responsibility and an independent life.
2. Procedures and treatment may have to be carried out in the absence of the patient's informed consent where he (or she) lacks the capacity to understand or express his wishes or is prevented by the mental illness from recognizing the threat to himself or others caused by his behaviour.
3. The psychiatrist's counter-transference i.e. his own personal desires, feelings or prejudices must not be allowed to bias or interfere with his best management of a patient.

Specific Areas of Ethical Debate

Sterilization of Minors

Clear medical indications for sterilization may exist in malignant conditions of the genital organs or in treatment of severe injuries. The immediate needs of the patient are paramount and take priority. The hotly disputed area concerns requests for sterilization from parents or guardians or society for eugenic reasons (e.g. to prevent Huntington's chorea being reproduced) or for pregnancy prevention in the severely subnormal.

Gostin[4] quoted Ministry of Health figures for 1973 and 1974 disclosing that 38 teenagers had been sterilized, four being under sixteen years of age, and advocated a Bill of Rights to protect such patients and a committee, with lay representation, to consider each case. The doctors involved may be moved with compassion but the ethical principles must take account of the patient's rights and future wishes, the unknown potential for improvement and the degree of risk must be balanced against the psychic and operative trauma. Perhaps a way out will be provided by better reversible birth control methods which do not depend on intellect and memory to use them effectively.

In such cases the doctor should make his judgment from the patient's viewpoint using his prognostic skills as far as possible. He should submit his views to the widest discussion with the parents, family doctor, paediatricians, social workers, teachers and other involved disciplines within the bounds of confidentiality. With all this, painful heart searching will still be necessary over individual decisions although in general terms the doctor will prefer not to interfere and will resist State-directed eugenic planning.

Sexual Expression

A mutually satisfying, heterosexual genital union in a stable relationship is the generally accepted aim of human maturity, but where disorders of sexual expression occur the doctor often has a difficult role to play. His attitude of concern and acceptance is what the patient most needs when he has become aware of his difficulties in sexual adjustment; the pain of feeling different and the consequent loneliness and isolation are acute. The heterosexually orientated doctor can provide much comfort in this way and be satisfied he is following Christ's example. He must not expect to be able to restore people whose damaged sexual adjustment has been fixed or declared in 'coming out' into a 'gay' society but he must be realistic in discussing mutually agreeable aims of therapy with the patient. He will be faced with the need to accept and understand people who are homosexual,[5] transvestite, exhibitionists, voyeurs and fetishists even when they espouse a way of life he regards as abnormal. The doctor will want to promote the fullest development of the patients' potential to choose his or her sexual role and to control and discipline his desires for the satisfaction and enjoyment of the loved 'other'. As a therapist he will have to battle with unhappy rigidity, limited power and poor motivation, which characterizes patients handicapped or crippled in an abnormal sexual role. Such patients fear the adventure of change.

The main ethical difficulty comes in the doctor's attitude to the conscious and determined behaviour, of a militant or flaunting nature, by a patient with homosexual or other abnormal sexual expression who is engaged in attempts to teach or draw other people into his or her way of life. Our laws no longer ban homosexual behaviour between consenting adults in private, but are correctly framed to restrain those who proselytize children and young people. The danger arises from vulnerability in adolescence when masturbation (loving oneself before being ready to love another) and homophile contacts are common, (and some would suggest normal), stages of development. The doctor would counsel a young person, distressed by the possibility of homosexual orientation, that love and affection (and even some degree of physical expression) are not in themselves abnormal and have a definite role in the development of gender identity, as in the father and son relationships. What *is* abnormal is for the patient to be taken over by sexual desires, of either sort, and so pre-occupying him for long periods and damaging the development of other relationships in vocation and in his sport. The acting out of such fantasies physically in casual and shallow relationships where no real care for the other person is felt or expressed is also unacceptable. The therapist could encourage an adolescent seeking guidance to discuss sexual development and try to enable the patient to make a responsible, informed choice during this fluid stage of development.

Recently a disturbing movement advocating the involvement of children in pornographic films and behaviour has arisen from homosexual and other pressure groups. At the moment such behaviour is illegal. Historically and clinically the evidence of harm to children from the premature exposure to sexual activity should convince all doctors that pressure to change the law is for selfish and perverted reasons and should be strongly resisted.

The Use of Drugs

Our pill-orientated society often expects doctors to be dispensers of happiness or tranquillity through drug prescriptions. When confronted, a doctor's moral understanding and view of normality have to help him decide when the patient's complaints are due to relationships which are distorted and the patient is being dishonest to his own code of beliefs. The doctor's role (described by O. Hobart Mowrer[6]) may be to confront the patient with his self-deceit and encourage him to test this new integrity with those most important to him, his family, friends and neighbours.

In clinical practice, then, the doctor's decision to base the main therapeutic thrust on the social worker of the team by seeing the family together in their home may be reached by careful consideration, and would replace the usual medical model of doctor/patient contact to discuss drugs. Similarly, is it right for hypnotic drugs to be prescribed continuously rather than in short courses to cover crises? Even more doubtful is the long term, repeat prescription of minor tranquillizers. If the doctor believes that a 'brave new world' without pain or ecstasy, with Aldous Huxley's 'soma', is the future for mankind, then he will think it right to allow the use of such drugs. Is it not wiser, however, to start from the position that people can best concentrate on, resolve or accept their problems in a clear, undrugged state with a sympathetic listener alongside?

In the field of addiction to drugs or alcohol the ethically conservative doctor is in the paradoxical position of rejecting the condition and restraining the behaviour of the patient (e.g. drying out in hospital) but accepting, understanding and trying to rebuild the sufferer. Indeed, the patient needs to be reconciled with himself and helped before he can face his family and non-addicted friends because of the frequent depression which may follow drug withdrawal. The issue here is that ultimately only the patient can control his purposive behaviour to obtain and abuse illicit drugs or excess alcohol. Therefore, the therapist's resource must be encouraging, coercing, even manipulating situations so that the patient becomes free to change his ways.

The law makes a useful distinction between the addicted user of a drug who may be trapped and held by his habit and the addict who pushes supplies or initiates others. The latter is much more destructive and dangerous and terms of imprisonment are more frequently used for these offences. Sadly, the pressures of the drug scene may force the initiate to sell illicit drugs to pay for his own supply.

We need to consider critically the motivation of those eminent people who advocate the 'free pot' lobby and advise the removal of cannabis or hash smoking from the list of prohibited drugs. There is evidence of brain damage in heavy habitual smokers and a small but definite number of reports on the toxic psychoses precipitated by taking this drug. It is particularly destructive to University students or staff who take the edge off their intellectual capacity as the cost of temporary oblivion – and who never attain their working potential. The true response of the doctor is that he values drugs and uses them for defined conditions, giving specific instructions for clearly stated periods of time as indicated by the patient's need. Therefore, he will be cautious when prescribing powerful, potentially addictive drugs, such as heroin and barbiturates, which develop tolerance in a patient and tend towards increased dosage to provide equivalent effects. Even minor tranquillizers and the social use of alcohol and cigarettes can blur the perception and consciousness of an individual and thus fall short of the ideal. However, at these points, doctors are dealing with hurt, sick and broken people and, we need to recognize and accept the powerful social influences today supporting the misuse of drugs (see p. 123).

Private Psychotherapy

The high cost of psychoanalysis and psychotherapy, both as indi-viduals and in groups, has led to the National Health Service providing very restricted resources in this area. This is justified, firstly, because patients select themselves and need high motivation for change to benefit from psychotherapy. Secondly, there is the difficulty in showing the value of psychotherapy as a treatment because of the absence of a suitable yardstick of personal change and growth towards maturity. This has led some authors to attack the validity of regarding psychotherapy as a 'treatment' at all.[7] Others usefully examine the qualities of genuineness, empathy and warmth that characterize successful therapists.[8] The doctor involved in private practice must examine his ethical position when a patient is paying for regular sessions. What is his attitude to receiving payment and is it an important token of the patient's involvement and motivation or not?

Forensic Issues

The doctor called upon to give a psychiatric report to a Court of Law has a different relationship to a patient from the normal doctor/patient contract. He must make this clear to the patient and obtain written permission to give the confidential report before the interview.

Criminal behaviour and mental illness may co-exist without a causal relationship and the psychiatrist's task is to evaluate the patient's mental state at the time of the offence and to form an opinion of his intention if possible. For example, in cases of shoplifters evidence of present or past mental illness, especially depression, will be sought. Chronically psychotic (e.g. schizophrenic) patients are usually returned to the hospital by the police without being charged. The majority of shoplifters who have any mental disturbance are personality-disordered people reacting to acute crises in their lives. The psychiatrist may ethically bring these relevant, but otherwise confidential problems of the individual to the Court to enable the magistrate or judge to make a humane decision. It must be remembered by the doctor that a limited fine, a community service order or probation supervision may each be a way of respecting the individual's dignity in recognizing his responsibility for his acts even though there are extenuating circumstances. In this way the patient's internal self accusation and shame, which could lead to depressive guilt, may be avoided by the Court. The doctor should not feel that it is his task to 'get the patient off' even though this has been society's stereotype of the permissive psychiatrist. The psychiatrist is being asked to help the Court to handle the person by advising from his experience, his skill in interviewing and perhaps his provision of treatment facilities. This has led to the present discussion whether forensic psychiatry is a discipline of its own or a sub-speciality.

The integrity of the doctor may be tested when advising on the 'degree of dangerousness'[9] to society or its property represented by a mentally abnormal offender. Here the restraint of individual liberty may be at stake. Some violent patients, however, will welcome the security of Special Hospital or even locked units in mental hospitals, when they have insight into their destructive impulses and are afraid of being out of control of themselves. Should the Government's plans based on the Butler Report[10] be implemented by the creation of Regional Secure Units, perhaps the wider range of facilities for restraint and treatment will help the doctor's aim of avoiding custodial care and the institutionalization which can degrade human beings.

In other parts of the world reports that totalitarian regimes have abused psychiatric practice in order to torture or detain people who disagree politically with the regime, but who are not mentally ill, has caused the Royal College of Psychiatry to declare its rejection of such behaviour. The World Psychiatric Association Declaration of Hawaii (1977) (see p. 197) clarifies an acceptable position in this situation. The young doctor could be guided by these principles if asked to give an opinion on the right methods of questioning an imprisoned person or where fitness for punishment was being queried.

Physical Treatments

Electroconvulsive therapy (ECT) has been established as an effective treatment since its introduction in the 1930s. It is the quickest way to relieve the deep suffering of severe depressive illnesses and is especially effective in suicidal conditions and where retardation has stopped a patient eating and drinking. ECT is superior to other forms of treatment in severe puerperal psychoses and in hypomanic illnesses failing to respond to drugs. A few cases of schizophrenia where affective or catatonic features predominate also respond to ECT. It may be regarded as unethical or even negligent to withhold such a treatment out of prejudice when dealing with such patients.

The current attack on ECT, including a parliamentary attempt to ban it, arises from ignorance of the terrible experience of depression and the efficacy of ECT in terminating illness. However, this alarm has been raised in two ways. First, unreasoned and prejudiced attacks have occurred from several sources by those who perhaps wish to divert attention from their own doubtful techniques which suggest brainwashing. Second, there has been a real concern about the damage caused by too frequent use of ECT resulting in permanent loss of memory and brain damage. The ethical guidance, then, is to learn to use a powerful, effective treatment properly. A modified ECT technique, applied two or three times a week, under general anaesthesia with the use of short-acting muscle relaxants is safe. Used in this way it is safer than tooth extraction under general anaesthesia. In certain right-handed people unilateral application of the electrodes to the non-dominant hemisphere will further minimize the normal short-term memory loss, usually restricted to a few weeks, although the black experience of the illness may be thankfully obliterated. ECT courses are usually 6–8 treatments with 10 or 12 being given occasionally. The damage mentioned above arises only from prolonged and repeated courses of 20 daily applications often while the subject is maintained under modified narcosis.

Psychosurgical procedures to control or alter violent or unacceptable behaviour raise strong emotions and tend to polarize opinions along prejudiced lines. The doctor needs to keep his mind open to the views of those skilled neurologists, neurosurgeons and psychiatrists, who, working with leucotomy and similar operations, are sincerely attempting to help very damaged patients. Equally those involved in psychosurgery need to listen to the concern expressed by private individuals, and to the religious point of view. Man's nature has a spiritual dimension and there is in him the potential for change and healing without the need for resorting to destructive remedies.

Leucotomy arose from Egas Moniz's work on chimpanzees in the 1930s and became over-used as a treatment for schizophrenia in the 1950s before the discovery of chlorpromazine which led to the first effective therapy. Nowadays, modified, stereotactic techniques minimize the personality defects caused by the earlier standard operations. The current indications are severe obsessional neuroses, severe, recurrent life-threatening depressive illnesses and chronic tension states.

Leucotomy is contra-indicated in most psychotic illnesses and in personality disorders where defective impulse-control has led to violence and destructiveness because one result of the operation is to lessen the inhibitions and this could make the problem worse. Another ethical problem confronting the psychiatrist lies in the difficulty of obtaining 'informed consent' from a frightened, ill patient and his relatives. Without a clear explanation of the operative procedure, the rehabilitation which must follow and the possible benefits and risks involved, a doctor should hesitate to carry out an irreversible brain operation.

Recent moves to restrict psychosurgery to special centres under the control of a mixed committee may increase the chance of balanced decisions. These would include clinicians not involved with the neurosurgical and psychiatric team as well as legal, administrative and lay members. Is it too much to hope that decisions on each individual case would only be reached after committee members had met the patient and his relatives privately?

Multidisciplinary Teams

Through the Hospital Advisory Service and the reports of other enquiries into large mental hospitals it has emerged that the Therapeutic Community aims, pioneered by such men as Denis Martin,[11] Maxwell Jones[12] and David Clark,[13] are important in preventing institutions from degrading patients. These principles involved lifting physical restraints, opening locked doors and giving psychiatric patients freedom and opportunity to express their views with staff and patients working together towards a therapeutic relationship. Behind the pioneering of these ideals was a Christian view of man: that he can be reconciled to himself and others by an honest and open sharing, by forgiveness leading to acceptance and by a new maturity and responsibility for his actions. Ethically this produces no problem because all modern treatments can be carried out in such a therapeutic milieu. The two difficult problems are first confidentiality and second ultimate responsibility. Both arise from the stress of working as a team composed of many disciplines including doctors, nurses, social workers, psychologists, occupational and other activity therapists.

If all staff members contribute from their different skills and fulfil their role in the team, the patient should feel confident that everyone is trying to help him and can be trusted with his secrets. In addition, the psychiatrist gains important information from the views of other disciplines and often treatment is delegated to individual staff members who are especially equipped to help a particular patient. Ultimately, however, the doctor is clinically responsible for the work of his colleagues in the care of patients and he must know them individually. He must be accessible to them to share difficulties, and be prepared to stand with them when things go wrong. A doctor working this way needs a secure ethical foundation and the courage to share himself with his team. A true religious faith gives him an advantage in this situation, particularly if he finds there is a consistency of ethical understanding in his team.

The Future

In conclusion psychiatry, as a modern medical speciality, is only thirty years old. The rapid advances in biochemistry are likely to be linked with an increasing number of active drugs. For this reason the young doctor must ensure that his treatment does not obscure the human distress. The changing structure of our society will probably continue to increase the stresses on our people. Those doctors who hold to the Judaeo-Christian position are able to base their teaching on the benefits of strong family life. The psychiatrist is trainer and superviser of other disciplines. Under his supervision laymen brought in as counsellors can both support and encourage people who are distressed to the point of breakdown: they have also a part to play in rehabilitation of patients after psychiatric treatment.

References

1. Mental Health Act (1959) London, HMSO.
2. Gostin, L. O. *A Human Condition – The MHA 1959–75*. London, NAMH.
3. Szasz, T. (1972) *The Myth of Mental Illness*. London, Paladin.
4. Gostin, L. O. *Op. cit.*
5. Moss, R. (1977) *Christians and Homosexuality*. Exeter, Paternoster Press.
6. Mowrer, O. Hobart. (1961) *Crisis in Religion & Psychiatry*. New York, Van Nostrand, Reinhold.
7. Szasz, T. *Op. cit.*
8. Truax, C. B. *et al.* (1966) Therapist empathy, genuineness and warmth and patient therapeutic outcome. *Journal of Consultative Psychology*, **30**, 395.

9. Scott, P. D. (1977) Assessing dangerousness in criminals. *British Journal of Psychiatry*, **131**, 127.
10. DHSS (1975) Mentally Abnormal Offenders. London, HMSO.
11. Martin, D. (1962) *Adventure in Psychiatry*. Oxford, Bruno Cassirer.
12. Jones, Maxwell (1968) *Social Psychiatry in Practice*. Harmondsworth, Penguin Books.
13. Clark, D. H. (1964) *Administrative Therapy*. London, Tavistock.

10

Safeguards in Clinical Research
David Tyrrell

Medicine has always been a learned profession. A great deal of time is taken in imparting essential knowledge to students before they practise and in trying to ensure that, once qualified, they stay abreast of medical knowledge for the rest of their professional lives. All this knowledge has to come from somewhere, and nowadays a great deal of it comes from clinical research. The conduct of clinical research brings up a number of ethical problems which are not encountered in other branches of medical practice, and it is an emotive subject about which many people are ill-informed.

In this chapter we shall see first of all how clinical research has developed over the centuries, and why it is intrinsically different from clinical care or preventive medicine. Then we shall mention briefly some of the evil things done in Nazi Germany in the name of research and the historic statements which were made in order to try and ensure that they did not happen again. Finally, we shall look at the difficult problem of translating general ethical ideas into sensible decisions about individual research projects and individual people.

The Growth of Clinical Research

Reading a history of medicine one realizes that for centuries the growth of medical knowledge was very slow and one of the objects of the Hippocratic Oath was, it seems, to ensure that doctors took note of what experienced older men said and themselves passed it on to others. The best doctors have been very acute observers of their patients, and many early advances in medicine were the result of observations on one or more patients with careful analysis of the records – most diseases were first recognized in this way. But in addition there has always been an experimental aspect to medical care, that of therapy. In most cases one cannot be really certain how a patient will respond to medical treatment or to an operation; one balances in one's mind the risk of doing nothing (the prognosis of the untreated disease) against the probability of success or harmful effects if one or other line of treatment is taken. Thus clinical observation, and the trials of therapy are both as old as medicine itself and both are covered by the ethics of medical care. Clinical enquiry is needed anyway before treatment can be considered, and its subsequent analysis will not affect the patient. The doctor trying a new treatment does so in the hope of helping the patient more than he could with previous treatments, and there can be nothing ethically wrong with that.

Much clinical research still falls within these two categories, although methods have changed considerably over the centuries. After history-taking and physical examination the modern patient undergoes numerous investigations, biochemical, electrical, radiological and so on, and these involve discomfort and sometimes risk. The doctor who decides to order such investigations makes a decision with an ethical aspect to it – that in order to have the greatest hope of treating the patient successfully he should have the additional information provided by these investigations, in spite of the discomfort and risk involved. This is a problem of the use of investigation in clinical care rather than clinical research and we shall not pursue it further here, though the results obtained may be used for research.

Controlled Trials

The second category, trials of treatment, has undergone considerable change in recent years because of the introduction of the controlled trial. The ethical problems this presents are inseparable from the logical and scientific reasons for the investigation. Those who oppose such trials assert that half the patients will be denied treatment, that the patient and doctor will never know whether they are treated or not, and that the decision on whether a patient is treated will be a matter of chance. The basic reason for developing the controlled trial is that patients and their illnesses are very variable and it is often difficult to decide whether they are getting better or not and whether any improvement is due to the treatment they have been given.

These difficulties can be overcome in the following way. First of all the response of treated patients is compared with that of untreated patients. In the past this was done retrospectively, that is to say a physician might compare the fate of patients with septicaemia who had been treated with penicillin with that of a previous series of patients who had not. The result is quite clear – those with penicillin-sensitive organisms usually survive, whereas most of the untreated patients die, and it can be concluded that the treatment is effective. It is just possible that the sort of bacteria or the sort of patient changed just when the physician started using the treatment and that this is responsible for the better results, but it is very unlikely. However, it is rare these days to see dramatic effects like this. Improvements which occur are likely to be small, and to detect these with certainty it is necessary to divide patients into groups and to observe and manage the untreated patients under exactly the same conditions as those who are treated. In order to avoid bias in the selection of patients for treatment, those who are to be treated are chosen by some impartial method, such as whether they were born on an odd or even date, or the use of random numbers. In order to avoid bias in the observation of the results of treatment neither the patients nor the doctor must know who is being treated and therefore the untreated patients are given tablets (placebo) or other medicaments which look exactly like the active treatment under test – this procedure is called a 'placebo-controlled double blind therapeutic trial'.

Whether this is ethical or not depends firstly on whether a proper comparison is being made. If it is known, to use our previous example, that penicillin does cure septicaemia, it will never be right in this disease to conduct a placebo-controlled trial with a new antibiotic in order to answer the question 'Is the new drug treatment better than no treatment?', because that would mean denying some patients treatment which would be almost certain to benefit them. On the other hand if a new antibiotic becomes available which, as a result of laboratory and animal tests, shows promise of being better than penicillin, it would be right to do a comparative trial of the new antibiotic with penicillin, in which the control group would have penicillin, rather than the placebo, and the results should answer the question, 'Is the new antibiotic better than penicillin treatment?'.

These examples illustrate two situations in which double-blind trials are needed – if there is no effective treatment for a condition and a preliminary trial shows no startling benefit from a new treatment, a placebo-controlled trial is needed to answer the question, 'Does the treatment do any good?'. If a possible improvement on a standard treatment is suggested, there is need for a comparative trial to answer the question, 'Is the new treatment better than the best available treatment?'. In these circumstances the patient is getting either a treatment which *may* do him good, when nothing else will, or else the best available treatment or something which *may* be better. Of course, there may not be agreement on the current state of knowledge – for example, whether the new treatment *does* seem better than the current treatment, or exactly what the best current treatment is. Thus two people, equally anxious to perform an ethical study, could hold opposite views on whether or not a trial was justifiable. It would not be possible to get an absolute ruling on who was right, though one could probably get a majority view by consulting others who had expert knowledge of the field of science involved.

Experiments on Humans

An important type of clinical research in use today is experimentation on healthy human beings. This was rare in the past, though John Hunter proved that venereal disease was infectious by inoculating himself with infected discharges. In recent years large numbers of volunteers have been inoculated with other infectious materials – thousands have been to the Common Cold Unit alone – and thousands more have taken chemicals of various sorts in order that their general pharmacological effects may be observed. Other volunteers have been used in physiological experiments, for example to study the effect of exercise on the circulation or of pain on the excretion of urine. These experiments may have many ethical problems similar to those in the previous examples, such as whether there is any risk in measuring the circulatory response, for example by passing a cardiac catheter, and whether control subjects are needed. In one respect however the whole situation is completely different and this can be illustrated in the following way. When a person feels ill he comes to the doctor and either explicitly or by implication enters into an agreement with him which can be summarized by the little conversation reproduced as Table 10.1.

Table 10.1 *The doctor-patient relationship*

Patient: I feel ill. Please make me better.
Doctor: I will do my best, but I may hurt you and I cannot guarantee success.
Patient: That's alright, but I assume everything you do will be done either to make a diagnosis or to cure my disease.

In the case of someone who becomes a volunteer the initiative comes from the doctor or scientist who wishes to perform the experiment and the relationship between them may be expressed in terms of a different conversation reproduced as Table 10.2.

Table 10.2 *The doctor-volunteer relationship*

Doctor: I want to do an experiment. Will you help me?
Volunteer: Provided you explain what it's all about and what will happen to me.
Doctor: I shall be glad to do so. The experiment is needed to answer an important scientific question and it won't do you any harm.
Volunteer: I agree for now – though I may change my mind later.

It is generally agreed that the responsibility for the safety and well-being of the volunteer is that of the doctor, and if anything goes wrong, even if there is no evidence that he was negligent, it is the responsibility of the doctor and the organization supporting him to compensate the volunteer in whatever way may be appropriate. The organization may meet such claims from its own resources or it may take out insurance for the purpose.

There are occasions when someone in hospital may be both a patient and a volunteer and then difficulties and misunderstandings can quite easily occur. For example, a man may be admitted to hospital with a condition, the cause of which is not understood. In order to test a theory about the cause of the disease, or some other aspect of it, the doctor may wish to perform some investigation which is not required either for the diagnosis or for the treatment, and the results obtained cannot possibly help in the patient's case. If such investigation is performed without comment the patient will assume, as in Table 1, that it is being done for his benefit whereas really it is done to satisfy the doctor's curiosity, and the patient has been deceived. The correct thing to do is obviously to have a conversation with the patient along the line of Table 2. This is the significance of the procedure of obtaining the patient's consent before beginning to conduct research on him. 'Informed consent' is the American term and 'true consent' is that of the British MRC. These two phrases emphasize two important points about the consent – firstly that the individual understands within the limits of his education and the research worker's knowledge, what is being asked of him and what may happen, and secondly that he understands that he has a genuine choice – he does not have to agree. We shall return to the problem of the patient's consent later, but it is worth noting here that there are difficulties with the concept. As the information available even to the doctor is incomplete there is really no such thing as fully informed consent so 'true consent' is the better term.

The Nuremberg Trials and After

After World War II there were protracted legal proceedings at Nuremberg at which surviving Nazi officials were tried for their part in War Crimes of various sorts. Among these were cases of experiments on human beings which horrified the civilized world. They included the intravenous injection of phenol into inmates of concentration camps in order to study its lethal effect and the infection of other subjects with typhus. Not only was there no question of asking consent, but the procedures were almost uniformly fatal, and it was generally thought that the standards of experimental design and observation were very poor, so that little information of value was obtained. Naturally this evoked a strong reaction and under the present law it is virtually impossible to conduct experiments of any sort on human beings in West Germany. Elsewhere reactions were less strict but the World Medical Association's Helsinki Declaration (see Appendix, p. 193) made it clear that any experiment which had an appreciable risk of doing any harm to a patient was not to be allowed and that the patient's permission was always to be obtained before anything was done to him. The Medical Research Council of Britain also issued a much quoted and similar statement on experiments in human beings (p. 150) and indicated the sort of safeguards which they expected would be observed.

There have been two subsequent reports of perversions of clinical research like those described at Nuremberg; Beecher in the USA and Pappworth in Britain have drawn attention to experiments, mostly reported in the scientific literature, in which milder, but neverthe-less undesirable and unethical experiments had been performed. The generally more critical atmosphere, of which these publications are an example, led to the Royal College of Physicians setting up a committee to discuss the supervision of the ethics of clinical investig-ation in institutions. Arising from its recommendations came the decision to set up ethical committees (sometimes called Research Ethical Committees) which had the strong backing of the Depart-ment of Health. Such committees now exist in almost all hospitals where research is carried out. Review Committees with similar func-tions are also operating in centres of medical research in the USA.

An Ethical Committee System

As I know of no general review of practice in different centres, I shall describe in some detail the administrative arrangements used at Northwick Park Hospital, Harrow, to implement the sort of ethical checks which are needed to safeguard those who conduct experiments and to avoid those procedures that are unethical. This Committee has dealt with applications for hundreds of projects dealing with thousands of patients.

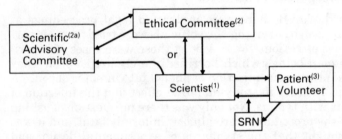

Fig. 10.1 The administrative arrangements in outline form.

The key group is the Ethical Committee which consists of
a) five hospital consultants who are not closely involved in research and a member of the junior medical staff,
b) the Chief Nursing Officer,
c) two General Practitioners from the area,
d) a lay member of the Area Health Authority.
A member of the Hospital Secretariat attends and also the Chair-man of the Scientific Advisory Group. A minimum number of consultants must be present to form a quorum.

The system operates as follows. A research worker, who may or may not be medically qualified, decides to submit an application to the Ethical Committee to conduct an experiment he has in mind. (This is not compulsory but the Hospital Authorities are not willing to support those who do experiments without Ethical Committee approval if subsequent difficulties or criticism are encountered.) The worker may apply by means of a letter, but usually he completes a form which will provide answers to the question which the Committee always asks. Notes on the back of the form indicate some of the general views of the Committee (see p. 150).

The form is sent to the Ethical Committee which immediately refers the project to the Scientific Advisory Committee, which looks at it from the scientific point of view, asking questions such as 'Is this intended to answer an important or a trivial question? Has it been done already, or could it be done in animals? Are the methods appropriate? Are the patients likely to be available? Are there likely to be unpleasant or dangerous effects for the volunteers?' The Advisory Committee Chairman is present at the next meeting of the main Committee who consider the project more broadly. First, on the basis of their own knowledge and that of their advisers they decide whether there is any substantial risk to volunteers, in which case they would not support it. If the study is poorly designed and could not give valid significant results, it would not be approved even if the procedures involved were simple. A guiding axiom is, 'Even a venepuncture without a good scientific reason is unethical'. Votes are not taken but projects are only approved when there is general assent.

If the project is approved the scientist would be told so, and at that time he may also be told of any reservations that the Committee has. He is then free to approach a volunteer, which he does in the presence of a witness who is a registered nurse. It is believed that a nurse will look after the patient's interests (with whom she has a direct link) since her main task is his care and her training enables her to understand in principle what the project is about, and to know whether the patient has been given an adequate explanation. If she agrees, and the volunteer consents, she signs to this effect on the sheet which records the research projects in which the patient is taking part. (In other centres the patient signs a consent form, but this provides no legal defence if something goes wrong and does not provide any means of checking how well the patient has understood the proposal. In the USA patients may be asked to sign a document of several pages which gives in some detail the plan of the study, the nature of all the procedures and any adverse effects which are likely to occur.) In the case of non-medically qualified scientists and of qualified doctors who wish to approach patients under the care of their colleagues, it is of course usual to obtain the approval of the doctor in charge before approaching a patient.

There is some concern about whether it is right for an Ethical Committee to supervise the experiments. Critics say that proceedings such as we have described are only 'whitewash', since after the meeting the scientist can go away and do what he likes. This is certainly true to some extent and the best safeguard now, as it always has been, is the sensitivity and honesty of the scientist involved. Nevertheless it is bad administrative practice to set up an organization which can direct that things be done without any means of ascertaining that they are. As there is a general distaste by professional people for reviewing personally the work of their colleagues, a limited degree of supervision has been arranged. This consists of a brief report on the progress of the investigation each half year from the research workers, and a responsibility placed on the nursing staff to report to the Chief Nursing Officer if they are concerned about what is happening to a patient involved in a research programme.

A more remote and later type of monitoring of research is provided by the medical journals in which the results of such research are eventually published. The papers submitted are usually sent to anonymous referees who are well able to make frank and trenchant criticism of both scientific and ethical aspects of the investigation. Furthermore it is common editorial policy to require that an author states specifically that the work was reviewed and approved by an ethical committee and that the consent of the patient was obtained. Since negative results are obtained at virtually the same human cost as positive results it is desirable that, for ethical reasons, such results are published so that they are not repeated unnecessarily by a research worker who is unaware of them. However for good scientific reasons this may not always happen.

Balancing Risks against Objectives

There are those who say that one should never take risks or even cause discomfort to normal subjects or to patients in the cause of science, but the advance of medicine depends upon the acceptance of such risks and discomforts. There is therefore a real or potential conflict between the advance of a science which will be able to help sick people and therefore is regarded as good, on the one hand, and doubts about the rights and wrongs of achieving that end by means of human experiment on the other.

It has been said that what little scientific knowledge was obtained by the Nazis should never be used because it was obtained in such a terrible way; not merely does the end not justify the means, but the use of such means pollutes the end obtained. One has sympathy with the emotions which lie behind such a view, but it should not be allowed to cloud the issue of whether human experiments under the rules of an ethical committee are right or not. It seems to be more reasonable to say that if a person in a free society can choose to do dangerous and uncomfortable things, like mountaineering or skin diving, for his own pleasure or health, he shall be at liberty to undertake similar risks and discomforts for the sake of knowledge which may benefit the practice of medicine.

There remain two difficulties, one related to 'true' and one to 'informed' consent. We have dealt with the problem of the normal adult patient, but children and those with impaired mental faculties cannot understand the choice being offered, and a common view in Britain is therefore that experimental studies which cannot benefit a child cannot be done within the law. However, for some mild investigations, such as collection of urine or blood, relatives or other responsible people do give permission for studies on mentally defective or mentally ill patients. The legal position has been re-examined recently and it has now been stated that a parent does have the right to consent to a procedure which does not benefit his child but may further some other good cause. However, the debate continues and we cannot yet see where it will end. In the past much research was done on servicemen and prisoners in the USA, but adults under strong discipline are not regarded in the UK as being suitable volunteers for medical research because they may not be able to give free and valid consent. There is even reluctance among some to accept students, for similar reasons! Volunteers are sometimes paid and this can also influence the ethical situation. It is normal and reasonable to recompense them for fares and other expenses, but excessive payment could act as a bribe and persuade a volunteer to take risks which he would not otherwise do.

The second difficulty is that no volunteer can really understand whether the experiment proposed is a good one with a worthwhile end in view. In this respect the introduction of an Ethical Committee is a very useful advance for it ensures that some sort of peer review takes place; in other words it makes sure that a scientist's ideas of what is a reasonable experiment appear so to others with similar expertise. This of course makes demands on those who make the review – they must not steal his ideas, his most valuable stock-in-trade, or divulge them to anyone else.

It is interesting that a great variety of people of various religions and of none can come to very similar views regarding the ethics of a proposed piece of work. It seems a very difficult and non-objective thing to do – to balance the 'worthwhileness' of a piece of research against the 'inconvenience or discomfort' to the volunteers involved, and yet it can be done just as we make decisions about whether it is right to expose children to the risk of falling in order that they may learn to walk, or learn self-reliance on a mountain. People of all types seem to have in common a very high regard for the volunteer; he is a fellow human being to be treated as they would like to be treated in his position, entitled to have the facts laid before him clearly and honestly and to be allowed to make up his mind freely whether to co-operate or not. Those with a lower opinion of man would be impatient of such 'overscrupulousness'; the majority would find it difficult to agree with them even though they could not say where their high regard for man came from or give reasons to justify it. We can be thankful that this concern is present and that it affects the practice of clinical research.

Appendix I   *Responsibility in Investigations on Human Subjects*, from the Report of the Medical Research Council for 1962–63 pp 21–25.
This Report draws attention to the increase in scientific investigation in modern medical practice. It discusses the use of new procedures in the investigation and treatment of the patient, controlled clinical trials and consent from those who volunteer for a specified form of investigation. Emphasis is placed upon the moral responsibility and professional discipline required from those who initiate, undertake or sponsor such research.

Appendix II   *Proposal for Research Project*. Brent and Harrow Area Health Authority, Northwick Park Hospital.
This is a form to be completed by an investigator, working at that hospital, who wishes to undertake a specific research project in the hospital involving work with human subjects. Notes of advice are given, together with an explanation of how the Ethical Committee does its work and how it should be approached.
The investigator is asked to give information on the objective of his proposed study, its design, the scientific background, the subjects and controls needed and the details of the procedures to which they will be submitted. The form is then given to the Ethical Committee for its consideration.

Further Reading

Beecher, H. K. (1966) Ethics and clinical research. *New England Journal of Medicine*, **274**, 1354–1360.
Duncan, A. S., Dunstan, G. R. & Welbourn, R. B. (Eds.) (1977) *Dictionary of Medical Ethics*. London, Darton, Longman & Todd. *See* articles on Clinical Trials, Consent, Human Experiment, Research Ethical Committees, Medical Research Council, etc.
Pappworth, M. H. (1967) *Human guinea pigs. Experimentation in man*. London, Routledge and Kegan Paul.
Reiser, S. J., Dyck, A. J. & Curran, W. J. (1977) *Ethics in Medicine: Historical Perspectives and Contemporary Concerns*. Cambridge, Mass., M.I.T. Press.

11

The Impact of Financial Constraint
Antony Wing

The economic realities of the cost of health care are making a new but inescapable challenge to medical ethics. It is no longer possible for doctors to take clinical decisions without taking some account of the resources which those decisions commit.[1] Care of suffering has always cost the concern of the healthier members of the community, but scientific medicine and almost unlimited possibilities for therapeutic intervention have escalated the price of compassion.

Expenditure on Health

The remorseless increase in expenditure on health needs is the reason for the present dilemma. The increase is best shown as the proportion of national incomes (as measured by gross national product (GNP)) spent on health but it is greater in terms of real money because the economies have been expanding (Table 11.1). In some countries, for example, USA, France and Western Germany, the proportion of GNP spent on health care has doubled in the last two decades.

Table 11.1 *Health Care Expenditures (Public & Private) as a percentage of GNP**

	West Germany	Sweden	USA	France	Canada	UK	Australia
1950			4.6	2.9		4.1	
1960	4.5		5.2	4.0	5.3	3.9	5.0
1965	6.9	6.0*	5.9	4.9	6.0	4.3	5.2*
1970	7.6	7.6	7.2	5.5	7.0	4.9	5.4*
1975	9.2*	9.0	8.3	6.8	7.1	6.0	7.5

* Reproduced from Maxwell, R. (1977) *A Simple Man's Approach to Health Economics*, with the author's permission.

Maxwell (1975) and Abel-Smith (1976) have identified the main causes. First there has been a change in the pattern of disease. The early years of scientific medicine saw easy victories over communicable diseases and those associated with malnutrition. Now attention must be turned to chronic illness and handicap and conditions associated with ageing. The treatment of ischaemic heart disease, of degenerative arthropathy and of cancer is more expensive than that of pneumonia and boils.

151

Second, advances in medical technology have taken place, particularly in the acute hospital sector. Some of these advances have resulted in savings in other areas. For instance, fetal monitoring has reduced infant mortality and in all probability the incidence of birth damage and therefore of long term handicap.

Third, medical profession and public have rising expectations both of high technology medicine and surgery and also of what constitutes acceptable standards of care for the mentally ill, handicapped and elderly who have often been neglected in the past. Public conscience is concerned to express itself on these matters and litigation in some countries and complaints procedures in others force standards up.

Fourth, rising manpower costs have a marked effect on health expenditure because of the labour intensive nature of providing health care. Advances in methods of medical care have seldom resulted in manpower reduction. In the United Kingdom 4% of the working population is now involved in giving health care which makes the National Health Service rank as a major industry. Wages in the health sector have undergone a 'catching up' process in recent years and the contribution of voluntary or low paid labour has decreased.

Fifth, there has been the change in method of finance from direct payment by individuals to insurance and Government funding. Governments are gradually assuming an ever larger role, rationalization and legislation preceding direct responsibility for the medical services. In the United States, where two thirds of funding comes from individuals or insurance schemes, the market forces of free enterprise have resulted in inadequate services to some areas and population groupings and excessive overlap in others. Such inequalities are politically and also probably ethically unacceptable, but their elimination is costly.

Now that health budgets are approaching 10% of GNP in some countries an inevitable clash with other political priorities is occurring. There are signs that Governments are beginning to apply the brakes on health expenditure.[2] In the United Kingdom central control over expenditure on the National Health Service has been notably successful in containing costs. Policies have been so successful, in fact, that credibility in any semblance of comprehensive care is now threatened.

Control of expenditure can only be achieved at the cost of equity or quality of care or both. The ethical dilemma is acute. We cannot have the highest quality of plant and personnel and enough of both to share among all who need it. Priorities in economies and in planning must be decided by consultation. What constitutes 'good' medical practice and 'right' clinical decisions will be determined by cost effective analysis as well as by scientific correctness and by humanitarian content. The medical profession cannot turn a blind eye to these facts. It must find leaders who are prepared to grapple with the ethical impact of financial constraint.

Demand, Need and Resources

It is clear that not all experience of sickness results in the expression of a demand for medical services. Many people faced with symptoms within themselves deliberately take no action. Many others practise some form of self care. Thirty per cent of all drug sales by value are dispensed without a doctor's prescription (see p. 117).

Demand for medical services varies with social status. Medical consultations are more common among spinsters, widows and divorcees than among married women. Admissions to hospital occur more frequently among the families of manual workers than those of the professional classes. The elderly make most demands on medical services. The life-style of a society may potently augment its medical demands and expectations. An important determinant is the availability of resources. Long waiting lists, full consulting rooms, queues, all reduce demand.

It seems to us that it is at this point that Christian values of non-indulgent living, of mutually supportive family, church and community relationships and of self-help and reliance may counteract increasing dependency on and dominance by 'expert' medical professionals. Such an influence would be healthy.

Demand is controlled by the ethos of society; medical need can only be defined by medical opinion. If medicine has something useful to offer to the person who makes or should make a demand upon it then there is a need for resource to meet that opportunity for useful service. Casualty Departments must be provided to handle accidents, surgery must be available for acute abdominal emergencies, obstetric care for pregnant women. But what sophistication is required by these emergency services? How much back-up do they need? The need of resources may be a matter of fashion, and fashion is dictated by doctors.

Economists are beginning to look critically at doctors' demands for resources to meet medical needs. It has been shown that availability of beds determines the number of admissions and length of stay.[3] Medical assessment based on usage of resources has a relative value only; it is not an absolute measure of need. Experience in provision of curative facilities seems to indicate that needs expand to utilize the available resources.

Has the increased channelling of resources to meet rising health expenditure reduced the economic cost of ill health? Unfortunately, no. In the United Kingdom 16 working days were lost due to sickness per employed person in 1971. Sickness rates are rising with nervousness, debility and headache accounting for an increased proportion of certification. These causes are not exclusively medical but probably represent a behaviour pattern in response to modern working conditions and social pressures. Political expectation (which might now be thought to be naive) that an efficient health service would contribute to a contented and productive work force has not been fulfilled.

However, although Britain is a low spender on health care by comparison with other Western countries, many indicators of the nation's health, notably infant and other mortality statistics suggest that the limited resources are being used relatively wisely. Indeed by comparison with the high spending and poor mortality statistics of the United States drives us to the conclusion that spending more on health does not necessarily buy better health.

Allocation of Resources

The practical objections to permitting medical resources to be distributed according to the interplay of free market forces are becoming clear. The conventional market system of demand and supply is inappropriate because it is the doctor as supplier and not the patient as user who determines how resources shall be utilized and how much quantity and quality of care shall be given. Doctors therefore generate increased costs.[4] A free market for medical resources results in inequitable distribution with resources being concentrated in areas of high profitability to the neglect of areas of need and poverty. Awakening public conscience will not permit this to continue and government must begin to take steps to improve the services in deprived areas. As soon as this intervention begins the balance between supply and demand is disturbed and free market forces no longer exert any constraint on medical expenditure.

Inevitably health care provision becomes not only a matter for public concern but also for communal responsibility. Decisions about the organization of medical care and about priorities and the control of development and expenditure, namely rationing, are progressively translated into the political arena.[5]

High expense is concentrated in hospitals which consume most of the capital expenditure and more than 50% of revenue costs. In western countries approximately 100 beds are provided per 10,000 of population. The high cost of the hospital bed is forcing its more efficient usage. In many countries the number of beds is now gradually decreasing. The average length of in-patient stay is also decreasing and the throughput per hospital bed is rising.

Research into the optimal duration of in-patient treatment following myocardial infarction could have far reaching implications for medical economics.[6] Furthermore, the requirement for hospital admission for myocardial infarction has been questioned in a random controlled trial.[7] Because of high bed costs, economy may be better served by out patient tests, pre-planned investigations and multiple batches of tests ordered without waiting for previous results.

Intensive use of an acute hospital can result in an average length of stay of less than 11 days and, with an 85% bed occupancy, about 27 cases can be handled per bed per year. It has been estimated that if these figures, now regularly achieved in the United States, were reached in French hospitals then almost 50% of the capacity of the hospitals in that country could be closed.

It is unethical to allow parochial competition to result in duplication of specialized centres because the quality of clinical service falls off if insufficient workload is available. Thus heart surgery units with a low workload were found to have a higher mortality than centres used more intensively. Flexibility of plant and personnel is necessary to avoid waste of facilities when medical needs change. Excessive specialization of professional roles may therefore be both a hazard to the individual and an economic encumbrance. It is a supreme challenge to the ethical stance of a physician or surgeon when he must face up to the fact that skills acquired over the most productive years of his professional life no longer merit prestigious facilities. If these uncomfortable facts must be accepted by the profession, they must also be acknowledged by the trades union leadership of ancillary workers.

The ethics of good economy require that the acute hospital facility is not isolated but integrated efficiently into the rest of the health services. Costs of care in an acute hospital are three times those of a long stay unit and five times those of intensive home care. Thus the care of handicapped children by foster parents, liberally supported by financial allowances and community services, is half the cost of institutional care. Further, the occupation of beds in acute general hospitals by geriatric patients requiring long term care is inappropriate and blocks the more intensive use which should be made of high technology areas. It was hoped that re-organization of the administrative structure of the National Health Service so that institutional and community services were integrated at local level would help in matching the level of need with the appropriate level of resource. In the event cumbersome bureaucracy and financial stringency impeded the desired flexibility.

Methods of Cutting Costs

Good primary medical care prevents excessive and inappropriate use of specialist services. The activities of the whole primary care team prevent some patients' admission to hospital, and facilitate early discharge of others, thus reducing the use of expensive facilities. The team needs a base, a health centre from which to operate and within which to co-ordinate its members. The health centre is increasingly seen less as a casualty clearing station and more as a spearhead for the medical education of the community so that instincts for self care and for healthy living are developed at

community and family level. This approach has been notably successful in modern China where informed lay personnel are used as
educators. It is a useful way of developing preventive medical care
but, most important, it reduces pressure on the more expensive
aspects of health services.

Efficient use of hospital services can also be helped by cost effective
analysis of methods of treatment. For example, studies of alternative
methods of treating varicose veins – outpatient injection versus in-
patient stripping operations – have been carried out to test whether
the cheaper methods achieve as good clinical results.[8] True cost, of
course, must include some assessment of time away from work and of
the impact of the whole procedure on the patient's family and its
economy. If the design of the study is satisfactory and the cheaper
method is shown not to be inferior, there will be ethical pressure on
clinicians to adopt the resource sparing approach. It is ethically
incumbent on the profession to turn its attention in the direction of
such research projects to maximize the efficient use of resources. If
doctors do not respond imaginatively to financial pressures, they can
only anticipate increasing frustrations and curbs on their activities.

One method for encouraging economic thinking is the allocation of
defined budgets to areas, services and departments. The size of the
unit must be large enough for choices about priorities but small
enough for the members to identify personally with it. Fixed budgets
risk inflexibility and stagnation of development, but provide incentive to take decisions on economic grounds. Doctors recoil from having to cost quality of care, but who but they are better qualified to
attempt this value judgment? Decentralization of economic constraint seems less likely than centralized control to engender frustration. Some form of rationing of resources is inevitable. Careful
thought must be given to the ethical implications of how this is put
into effect. Nothing could be worse than heavy-handed treasury
curbs on caring endeavour. However, failure by the caring professions to accept the challenge of financial constraint would be equally
counter-productive.

As an inevitable accompaniment of resource limitation political
pressure has built up for a fair distribution of resources. The Resource
Allocation Working Party has devised ingenious formulae to take
account of differences in age structure and other demographic factors
affecting medical needs.[9] On this basis it is hoped gradually to redis-
tribute medical resources. It is difficult to apply these formulae at a
time of sharp financial restraint. To take from areas of relative
excellence and give to areas of relative deprivation may result only in
generalized mediocrity. The process can only be gradual and can only
be applied by organizing differential rates of growth and development so that a catching up process can occur. During this process it is
vital for the future of medical education and other professional training that centres where comparatively lavish resources have been

accumulated for purposes of education and research should not be dismembered out of consideration only for the service role of these centres. To do so would be to ration out the seed corn of the medical heritage of the United Kingdom. The ethics of redistribution require some attention to be paid to the long term future of medicine.

Contribution of Preventive Medicine

It is attractive to think that prevention of ill health will not only prevent suffering but reduce expenditure on medical cures and caring services.[10]

However, causes of ill health are often multifactorial involving living conditions, food habits, life styles and economic status. In a medical programme in rural Guatemala the attack on ill health dictated that curative medicine came low on the list of priorities after social and economic justice, land tenure, agricultural production and marketing, population control, malnutrition and health training.[11] In Western societies, there remain well known factors which have not been eliminated. Not enough is known about how to reduce smoking habits and how to prevent obesity.

It may be self evident that if elimination of primitive practice by the 'women of the village' in India will eliminate neonatal tetanus, then ruthless re-education must be pursued. However, more articulate obstruction to the eradication of cigarette smoking is encountered in so called 'advanced' cultures. Counteraction of the medical demands of alcoholism in France would also be likely to provoke voluble resistance.

These examples of how improvement in health can be achieved by education of the community make the point that many preventive measures do not consist in removing infective agents from the environment or in replacing dietary deficiencies or in a program of vaccination. They concern the current life style and the social and cultural history of society. The medical profession needs to see itself not only as a curer of ailments but as a healer in a fuller sense. Unfortunately preventive medicine often appears less exciting, challenging and rewarding than individual curative medicine and surgery. In Northern India a community health scheme which includes a large educational programme fires the enthusiasm of the best medical graduates.[12] The ethic taught to medical students of developed countries should also exalt the medical and social value of preventive endeavour and permit critical assessment of any massive use of resources for marginal improvements in disease therapy.

Commercial Exploitation

The pharmaceutical industry has made large profits out of medical prescribing and pharmaceutical companies consistently rank among the most profitable of industrial groups. The total value of world pharmaceutical sales was £7,000 million in 1970 and is expected to top £15,000 million by 1980. The ethic of large profits has been defended on grounds of the need to provide capital for further research and because of the 'risk-factor' of developing and marketing new drugs (see p. 119).

The industry spends heavily on sales promotion with advertising, promotional meetings, and sales representatives all aiming for the attention of the doctor. Annual promotion costs in the United Kingdom amounted to £33 million per year and at these rates it has been calculated that more will be spent advertising drugs to a doctor during his professional life than it costs to train him in the first place. However, many companies fully accept the important role which they play in continuing medical education and their sponsorship of scientific meetings, scientific journals and of research by academic departments must be acknowledged. Ethical problems arise when sponsorship seeks to take a controlling interest or advertising to misrepresent the results of research into drug action, making too much of marginal advantages over previous drugs and playing down side effects. The total cost of promotional budget poses the question of whether this expenditure is ethically defensible since it adds to the cost of patient therapy and this cost must also be paid in developing countries. Controls over profit margins are being introduced in some countries, and in others controls over the introduction of new drugs are beginning to be applied sensibly. Bulk purchasing and manufacturing under licence are further methods of keeping down the drug bill.

The individual doctor needs to be aware of the intense commercial pressures under which he practises. He will learn to concentrate his prescribing practice on small numbers of drugs for common conditions, to know their side effects and interactions, and to resist change in his practice unless there is a very good reason. Medical education can only inculcate responsible attitudes, for the prescriptions which a doctor writes during most of his professional life will be largely for drugs unknown when he was a medical student. It requires considerable personal discipline to recall official rather than brand names when writing prescriptions, to be wary of repeated prescriptions and not to prescribe excessive quantities.

Professional Remuneration

The method by which doctors are paid has an effect on the style of medical practice and on the cost of a medical service. Each of the methods has some ethical implications. The method of payment selected usually depends on previous methods employed in the country concerned.

Fee for item of service has its roots in the earliest forms of medical practice. Its worst effect is to create a barrier between the needy and possibly poor and uninsured patient and the medical treatment he requires. It does make the patient aware of the cost of what is being done to him. It also encourages the provision of modern, well equipped and efficiently staffed premises. Under health insurance or State financed schemes for re-imbursement it has an inflationary effect on total costs of health services. Fees are usually paid for procedures and this tends towards multiple consultations, prescriptions and injections and the performance of many investigations rather than encouraging observation and listening. Since specialists perform specialized procedures they earn more and excessive specialization and neglect of basic primary care may ensue. Surgery may be carried out by insufficiently experienced operators because of the attraction of the fee for the operation. Furthermore, urban practice is likely to be more remunerative and this does nothing to help in the distribution of medical resources. Payment by fee for item of service results in proliferation of controls, and price setting procedures. Litigation frequently accompanies this method of payment leading, in turn, to 'defensive' medicine characterized by heavy investigation and therefore extravagant use of resources.

Capitation fee payment is only applicable in the primary care area. The terms of service are designed so that the doctor does not accept responsibility for too large a list. Capitation fee encourages the distribution of doctors and does something to help continuity of care. However, although the capitation fee for the elderly may be larger, it does not always encourage taking on the care of difficult or demanding patients, nor the upgrading of practice premises. In fact, under both capitation and fee for service systems of payment there are no financial incentives to provide a higher quality of care.

A *salaried system of payment* permits merit to be rewarded by promotion and salary differentials can be used to fill posts in less attractive areas. It removes competition for patients and makes doctors more willing to work together in teams. This improves the development of services and professional communication and particularly promotes the organization of medical education. Salaried payment of clinicians who hold university posts is therefore widely practised in many countries. Remuneration of academic posts must always be by a salary adequate to ensure that the best of doctoring ability is attracted to teaching centres.

The disadvantages of a salaried system are that there is no financial incentive to the doctor to work hard and ambitious doctors may become concerned with acquiring 'merit' in the way of non-clinical activities such as political leadership and academic achievements which catch the limelight rather than by dedication to their patients. Not even totalitarian regimes have abolished private practice entirely and in non-totalitarian countries a residuum of private practice is treasured by the profession as a corrective against the excesses of state control possible in an exclusively salaried service. It is therefore likely that some mixture of salaried service and private practice will be found in most countries. The worst of this mixture is found where salaries are low and defined hours worked are short as in South America where double standards of medical practice result and those who cannot afford private fees are seriously disadvantaged.

Payment by salary probably puts the greatest challenge to the doctors' ethical behaviour. In countries where the traditions of ethical medical practice run high it probably results in less undesirable side effects on the use of resources and on standards of care.

Whatever method of remuneration a doctor works under, professional ethics restrain him from profiteering or from altering the standard or style of care he gives at the dictates of his own financial advantage. Nevertheless, the financial rewards are a motivating factor and the system of payment should be carefully selected both by profession and employer so that it promotes the best care of the patient, the best developments in the future of medicine and the best use of medical resources. In this way the medical profession will be regarded as disinterested and worthy of the trust of patients and worthy to be entrusted with the utilization of a large quantum of a nation's resources.

Dialysis and Transplantation: A Challenge to the Ethical Use of Resources

One of the author's personal experiences of financial constraints has been the treatment of end-stage renal disease. The replacement of kidney function by dialysis and renal transplantation was shown to be worthwhile medical treatment by the mid 1960s. The past decade has witnessed the varying rates of development of programmes in different countries to make the treatments available to all who may profit from them. It was sobering to analyse the results achieved by comparing the number of patients alive per million of population on both forms of therapy in 31 different countries. We found that the number treated correlated significantly with the per capita GNP in US dollars in each country (Fig. 11.1).

The overall constraint of economics is plain. The money which a country can afford on individual curative medicine depends on its economic productivity. Human life has a variable price tag.[13] The chances of a needy individual receiving treatment without which he will die depends on the wealth of the society into which he was born.

Doctors working in this field have been very aware of the high cost of their treatments. They have therefore grouped themselves in collaborative studies such as that organized by the Registration Committee of the European Dialysis and Transplant Association. They have done this in order to produce statistics of the results achieved.

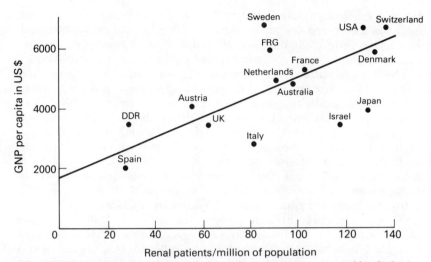

Fig. 11.1 Relationship between total number of patients treated by dialysis and transplantation per million of population and the per capita gross National Product in 15 different named countries. The regression line was drawn for data from 31 countries, r = 0.821 and is significant (P = <0.01). Figure reproduced from Wing, A. J., 1977. Prospects for the treatment of renal diseases, *British Medical Journal* 2, 881, with permission of the Editor.

Both the length of life-survival, and its quality of rehabilitation have been carefully assessed. No other treatment has been so comprehensively registered. Treatment achieves at least 55% survival at 5 years, which can be compared to 52% for the treatment of breast cancer, 15% for cancer of stomach, 21% for cancer of the lung, and 45% for coronary thrombosis in men aged 40–46 at onset. So far as the quality of life is concerned, 80% of transplanted or home dialysis patients are in full time employment and, presumably, paying taxes.

These results demonstrate the effectiveness of the treatment but the cost is high. It has been estimated that five years' hospital dialysis cost £50,000, five years' home dialysis £30,000 and five years of survival with a transplant £12,000. In the United States, where treatment threatened financial ruin of the patient who had to pay, a Congressional decision placed regular dialysis within the Medicare field, available as a right to all who need it. Detailed rules about reimbursement of physicians and of the contribution made by the patient resulted in an abrupt change in dialysis policy.[14] Home dialysis ceased to expand and highly efficient outpatient dialysis centres proliferated. The reverse effect has occurred in the UK due to very different economic pressures resulting from a different method of payment of physicians and of funding. Central control over the financing of developments in the National Health Service has prevented the growth in numbers of hospital centres in the UK and as a result physicians have had to press home dialysis till two thirds of all

UK dialysis patients are treating themselves at home. Pressure on facilities has forced doctors to deny treatment to patients who could neither perform home dialysis (often due to unsatisfactory domestic and family surroundings) nor be good subjects for transplantation.

These constraints have encouraged every technical innovation which may reduce the cost of treatment. Physicians have learned to resist the sales talk 'recommendations' of manufacturers of dialysers and to experiment with the re-use of 'disposable' equipment. Home dialysis, self help by patients and shortened schedules are all regularly practised to save costs. Inevitably a patient who would consume more than his 'fair share' of resources may be denied treatment. Thus selection in the UK has resulted in a younger average age of dialysis patients and a lower percentage of diabetics than in comparable countries such as France, Western Germany and Italy.

Because transplantation is cheaper, the Department of Health has taken much trouble in facilitating its organization, and stands financially firmly behind UK Transplant (an organ sharing organization) and promotes schemes to help organ procurement. This is welcomed by British physicians because of the rigours of home dialysis and because doctors do not lose financially if their patients opt for a transplant as a way out of dialysis. The growing concern not to miss kidneys suitable for grafting is resulting in some pressure on clinicians in intensive therapy units and neurosurgery centres to make organs available when brain death is diagnosed. Thus the cadaver kidney is seen as a valuable resource not to be squandered.

The treatment of end-stage renal disease powerfully indicates the ethical impact of financial constraint. It is I, the doctor, who must decide that some shall not live because in treating them I may jeopardize the therapy of others. A drug addict with renal failure is likely to be rejected from treatment, not because of any moralistic condemnation of his habits, but because he is a carrier of hepatitis B and thus threatens with closure the Renal Unit in which he is treated. I must create propaganda in my unit which puts pressure on patients not to get stuck on the limited hospital dialysis facilities but to submit themselves and their families to the incessant demands of home dialysis or to volunteer for transplantation. I must experiment with technology being willing to accept 'second best' and to make the value judgement that a certain price difference is not worth paying for a small gain in quality or safety.

The pressures under which I must dispose of our resources are increasingly common experience in medicine. The issues are particularly dramatic in this field because so much money is committed by clinical decisions and because the nature of these decisions is so often 'life or death'. We shall never stop trying to obtain increased resource allocation for our patients and will submit our results to scrutiny and, indeed, cost effective analysis and comparison with other clinical achievements.

In publicizing the appeal of these patients we have often become aware that they have a powerful public lobby because of their youth and critical need for treatment. Nevertheless, the only ethical course open to us is to press their claims to the limit, otherwise we fail the trust they place in us to be their advocates. At the end of the day we must accept the proportion of resources allocated for their care and by careful and economic organization do the best we can for as many as possible within the budget given us by Society. If we cannot treat all, then those left to die will be chosen because, in the opinions of doctors, they are likely to do less well on treatment than others.

Conclusion

If the medical and caring professions are to take their proper role in moulding decisions concerning the use of medical resources, then they must come to realize that financial constraint has an ethical impact. It forces the doctor to choose. Choice requires analysis of the cost effectiveness of medical and surgical endeavour and of the relative value of curative and preventive measures. Objective analysis and dispassionate choice is a challenge to ethical integrity. Factors which influence the motives of the doctor, notably the effect of his decision on his status and income, cannot be ignored. If doctors do not develop a method and ethic for choosing priorities in the face of economic pressures, then others will take the decisions for them. If the challenge is not accepted, professionalism will be sacrificed.

References

1. Owen, D. (1976) Clinical freedom and professional freedom. *Lancet*, **1**, 1006.
2. Mechanic, D. (1978) Approaches to controlling the costs of medical care. *New England Journal of Medicine*, **298**, 249.
3. Feldstein, M. S. (1968) *Economic Analysis for Health Service Efficiency.* Chicago, Markham.
4. Hiatt, H. H. (1977) Editorial: Lessons of the coronary by-pass debate. *New England Journal of Medicine*, **297**, 1462.
5. DHSS (1976) Priorities for Health and Personal Social Services in England: a consultative document. London, HMSO.
6. Ross, R. S. (1978) Editorial: Early discharge after heart attacks and the efficient use of hospitals. *New England Journal of Medicine*, **298**, 275.
7. Hill, J. D., Hampton, J. R. & Mitchell, J. R. A. (1978) A randomised trial of home versus hospital management for patients with suspected myocardial infarction. *Lancet*, **1**, 837.
8. Paichaud, D. & Weddell, J. M. The economics of treating varicose veins. *International Journal of Epidemiology*, **1**, 287.
9. DHSS (1976) Sharing of resources for health in England: Report of the Research Allocation Working Party. London, HMSO.
10. DHSS (1976) Prevention and health: everybody's business. London, HMSO.

11. Newell, K. W. (Ed.) (1975) *Health by the People*. Geneva, WHO.
12. Browne, S. G. (1977) The community health bandwagon comes to India. *World Medicine*, Oct. 19th, p. 93.
13. Card, W. I. & Mooney, G. H. (1977) What is the monetary value of a human life? *British Medical Journal*, 2, 1627.
14. Friedman, E. A. *et al.* (1978) Pragmatic realities in uremia therapy. *New England Journal of Medicine*, **298**, 368.
15. Wing, A. J. *et al.* (1978) Mortality and morbidity of re-using dialysers. *British Medical Journal*, 2, 853.

Further Reading

Abel-Smith, B. (1976) *Value for Money in Health Services*. London, Heinemann.
Berki, S. E. (1972) *Hospital Economics*. Lexington.
Bowen, R. A. (Ed.) (1974) Symposium Number 15, Constraints on the Advance of Medicine. *Proceedings of the Royal Society of Medicine*, **67**.
Cochrane, A. L. (1973) *Effectiveness and Efficiency*. London, Nuffield Provincial Hospitals Trust.
Cooper, M. H. (1975) *Rationing Health Care*. London, Croom Helm.
Douglas-Wilson, I. & McLachlan, C. (1973) *Health Service Prospects: an International Survey*. London, Nuffield Provincial Hospitals Trust.
Illich, I. (1975) *Medical Nemesis: The Expropriation of Health*. London, Calder and Boyers.
Maxwell, R. (1975) *Health Care: The Growing Dilemma*. A McKinsey survey report, 2nd Ed.
Phillips & Wolfe, (1978) *Clinical Practice and Economics*. London, Pitman Medical.
Reiser, E. S. J., Dyck, A. J. & Curran, W. J. (Eds.) (1977) *Ethics in Medicine: Historical Perspectives and Contemporary Concerns*. Cambridge, Mass., MIT Press.
Titmus, R. M. (1970) *The Gift Relationship: From Human Blood to Social Policy*. London, Allen & Unwin.

12

Preventive Medicine and Integration of Health Services
Stuart Horner

Preventive medicine has for many years been identified administratively and professionally with a separate group of doctors who have a specific responsibility for the prevention of disease within the community. Success has been spectacular far outweighing, in its impact on health, the achievements of curative medicine. Godber[1] has argued, however, that preventive medicine must use the skills of therapeutic medicine if further progress is to be made. The administrative separation of preventive medicine from the mainstream of health service practice was revoked by the reorganization of the National Health Service in 1974 and the emerging specialty of community medicine was then recognized.

The Faculty of Community Medicine, which was established in 1972, defined the specialty as 'that branch of medicine which deals with populations or groups rather than with individual patients. . . . It therefore comprises those doctors who try to measure accurately the needs of the population, both sick and well. It requires to bring to this study special knowledge of the principles of epidemiology, of the organization and evaluation of medical care systems, of the medical aspects of the administration of health services, and of the techniques of health education and rehabilitation which are comprised within the field of social and preventive medicine'.

Community physicians are, therefore, concerned with *all* aspects of the health care system, although the term 'community' is often misunderstood to relate only to medical care outside of hospitals. They deal with groups rather than with individual patients. They are also intimately involved in the management of health services[2] and provide medical advice to policy-forming bodies during the decision-making process.

The community physician has to face ethical problems different from those which arise during the care and treatment of individual patients and this includes some of the most topical and difficult issues of the present day. He will, of course, take the advice of colleagues, but he must usually make his decision alone without the continuing support which clinicians enjoy. The ethical problems he faces can be separated into three general categories: those affecting the individual and the community, those affecting his own personal views and standards, and those affecting his relations with his colleagues. Some questions have implications in all these areas.

The Individual and the Community

The problem of balancing the needs of the individual with the rights of society is not a new one. With the increasing interdependence among people and the growth of social care, the emphasis has been moving away from the individual towards the community and, indeed, towards the State. Some specific examples can be taken.

Infectious Diseases

In the latter part of the nineteenth century notification of infectious diseases to the new Medical Officers of Health was looked upon with grave misgivings because it was thought that the confidentiality of the doctor-patient relationship would thereby be broken. However, the value to the community in enabling outbreaks of infection to be identified, and in many cases controlled, was quickly realized, and this led to the compulsory notification of a large number of infectious diseases by the Act of 1899. The present list of notifiable diseases includes a number which are now so rare that specialized techniques of identification and public health control are essential and the confidential manner in which the information is handled serves in any case to remove much of the ground for this earlier objection. Few doctors today would advance ethical considerations as a reason for the current widespread under-notification of infectious diseases. The advantage has been clearly shown to lie with the needs of the community.

Renal Disease

The community physician is concerned with ethical problems arising from the provision of facilities for dialysis, either at hospital or in the home. Renal dialysis is costly[3] and the community physician knows that the management team, of which he is a member, has a fixed annual budget from which all health care requirements of the district must be met. The provision of every dialysis unit will reduce the resources available, for instance, for improvements in the accommodation of the elderly and the mentally handicapped or the prevention of ill-health in children. He has a duty to see that his clinical colleagues in dialysis units and those clinicians responsible for the individual clinical problems are brought into full discussion of all the issues involved before final decisions are taken. In such a situation there are real difficulties in balancing the needs of the individual with those of society. All individual needs cannot be sacrificed, and the community physician is under an obligation to deploy responsibly the resources that are available to him (see p. 153).

Fluoridation

The opponents of fluoridation of water supplies tended, initially, to cloud the ethical issues involved by abortive discussions on the real or imagined health hazards of the procedure. Recent discussion has concentrated on the issue of whether it constitutes mass medication. Doctors may themselves have contributed to this view by arguing that the *addition* of fluoride to that water would reduce the incidence of dental caries, implying the fluoridation is a therapeutic procedure. It might be more appropriate to regard dental caries as a deficiency disease and fluoridation as a correction of the deficiency on a community basis in the same way as thyroid disease, endemic in certain areas, has been largely eliminated by the addition of iodine to table salt. The fact that excessive intake of fluoride causes mottling of the teeth and, in extreme doses, other more serious medical problems, is not a criticism of the deficiency disease model any more than the ill-effects of overdosage of vitamin D mean that rickets is not a deficiency disease.

The ethical position is by no means clear. In view of the possibility of serious abuse, it seems clear that no doctor should accept the concept of mass treatment of disease by the therapeutic addition of substances to the diet of the individual without that person's knowledge or consent. On the other hand, it can equally be argued that no community should allow its members to suffer needless disease because of an intrinsic deficiency in their diet which could conveniently be remedied. While, therefore, mass medication should be rejected, a universal measure to restore the diet to that which is optimum for health is ethically acceptable even though an element of free choice is lost.

Immunization

There is also the need to balance the relative risks of the hazard itself with those of the preventive measure proposed. This is a problem which has arisen in particular with some immunization procedures. Knox[4] has recently discussed the concept of 'negligible risk to health'. In assessing the risks of contemporary living which individuals seem to accept and those which they reject, he discovered that a risk of one in 100,000 is apparently acceptable, but one in 10,000 is not. This can provide the community physician with an index by which he can judge the acceptability of a preventive measure against the health risk involved, on the assumption that such facts will eventually be presented to each individual involved. It also raises the ethical issue of whether the State has any right to accept and balance such risks on behalf of the individual. In the case of fluoridation, however, replacement of the deficiency is justified on the grounds that the procedure carries no risk. If a risk could be proved, even a negligible one, advice to community physicians would necessarily be very different.

Screening

Medical practice is based on an understanding by the patient that he is ill and that, if he wishes to be restored to health, he must seek out a particular doctor and follow his advice. Screening introduces a new element into this traditional relationship.

Doctors are taught (not always on reliable evidence) that the earlier a patient presents for treatment, the more likely it is to be successful. They are, therefore, conditioned to the concept of pre-symptomatic screening for disease. If patients can be identified before they themselves recognize that they are ill, then, it is argued, the disease process can be arrested at an early stage with an improved prognosis and long term economies in the costs of health care. Certainly the application of screening techniques to a number of diseases has led to a greater understanding of the processes involved, especially where the natural history of the disease is imperfectly understood. A study of the population of Bedford was made in an attempt to identify pre-symptomatic diabetes mellitus. It revealed a number of persons who had asymptomatic glycosuria and a continuing study is in progress to see whether treatment of these individuals prevents the long term complications of diabetes. Similarly, there is discussion as to whether carcinoma-*in situ* invariably leads to invasive carcinoma of the cervix – knowledge which is crucial to the continuation of the present national scheme for cervical smear testing.

The value of pre-symptomatic screening is discussed by Cochrane[5] and pre-occupation with this issue has tended to obscure the ethical implications of the change from the traditional doctor-patient relationship which is involved. In short, has the medical profession any responsibility for 'discovering' illness as distinct from responding to it when it presents? Illness which is seen by the doctor in the NHS is a very small proportion of the total illness within the community (Fig. 12.1). It is represented by those who die, together with those who are ill and who visit a doctor. There are, however, two other important groups. One, which could be four times as large as the number who attend a doctor,[6] comprises those who know that they are unwell but do not seek medical help and, the other, those who are ill but who do not yet know that they are ill. The total size of the two groups is not known but it could be very large, as the diagram indicates. The ethical dilemma lies in the fact that screening is likely to reveal significant numbers of ill people who do not at present seek medical help. If the doctor intervenes to discover illness without the patient making the first approach to him, the patient may legitimately argue that it is the doctor's responsibility also to provide effective treatment

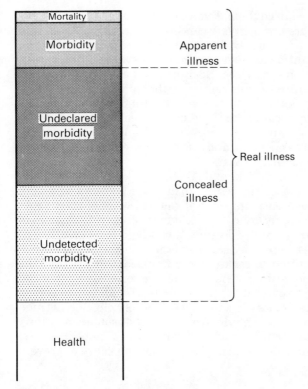

Fig. 12.1 The iceberg of disease.

for whatever is discovered. The medical profession could therefore find itself presented with a sum total of medically defined illness which, by its very size, it was quite unable to treat and for which the value of therapy had not yet been proved.

Moreover, might this transfer itself result in a gradual reduction in the perceived responsibility of the individual for his own health care? Such a trend would be most unfortunate at a time when the behaviour of the individual is being recognized as the most important aetiological factor in many of the most prevalent diseases in society.

Two illustrative examples will show that such an analysis is not as unreal as may at first appear. In the field of family planning a significant change in the attitude of society has occurred within a remarkably short time. Up to about ten years ago the planning of families was seen very much as a matter of individual responsibility. The concern of the Health Service was limited to the remedying of ignorance and to the provision of supplies. It was suggested, however, that the exercise of these functions did not always result in appropriate action by the individual. By an enabling Act in 1967 the emphasis changed and local health authorities were able to provide

services to all who required them. Even that was judged to be insufficient. 'Authorities' are now actively concerned to seek out those who
are at risk, that is, presumably, those who can be persuaded of the
need for family limitation and who, for one reason or another, choose
not to use the available services. Such people have been provided
with domiciliary facilities,[7] thus removing the final step of responsibility involved in making a visit to the local clinic. The next logical
step is compulsion (A parallel can be found in the situation regarding
abortion. With the progressive relaxation of legal restraints many
women are now offered abortion, and some may be encouraged to seek
it, just because the facilities exist.)

Secondly, the Chronic Sick and Disabled Persons Act, 1970,
imposed upon local authorities a duty to discover patients who were
handicapped. All such patients were of course aware of their problems and were, indeed, receiving medical care of varying degrees of
effectiveness from their family doctors. It was held to be insufficient
for local authorities to advertise services or make them widely available; they were required to seek out the handicapped whether the
latter wished to be identified or not. It must be seriously questioned
whether this should be carried to a point where a handicapped person
finds it difficult, if not impossible, to refuse offers of help. Such a trend
ought to be unacceptable in the Health Service, but some community
physicians may not have fully understood the ethical implications of
such activities in their laudable aim to further the cause of preventive medicine.

The Standards and Beliefs of the Community Physician

Provision of Services Contrary to Individual Ethical Beliefs

In recent years a number of legislative changes have been made
which have allowed the introduction of services which are contrary to
the beliefs and ethical standards of Christians. These pose special
problems to doctors appointed to advise authorities on the provision
of services such as, for example, contraception for the unmarried (see
p. 57) and abortion (see p. 64). The views of an individual clinician
should be known and understood by his colleagues and his patients, so
that those who do not like them may go (or be referred) elsewhere. He
does not then face an unnecessary conflict. In contrast the community physician may be giving advice to an Authority serving those of
many different ethical views and the Christian will find himself in a
minority position on certain issues. Moreover, he may find it difficult
to ascertain the wishes of the majority, who often go unheard, against
vocal, minority, pressure groups. This makes it all the more difficult
to decide whether or not he should support the provision of a service
with which he personally disagrees so that those who wish it may
benefit, and whether it is enough simply to state his own view and

then acquiesce in what he feels the majority require. He has a duty to assess the need as accurately as possible, to be aware of the dangers inherent in the methods of assessment in use, and be ready to criticize spurious statistics produced by activists on either side. Where a community physician is satisfied that there is a case for the introduction of a service, it would be unrealistic and inappropriate for him to oppose it, even though he disagreed with it on ethical grounds. It is not illogical for him, however, to continue to speak against a service although he may have reluctantly acquiesced in its implementation.

Health Education

The community physician is involved in health education either personally or through his responsibility for the work of professional health education officers.

Health education among children has moved away from a didactic approach and nowadays aims to present facts, leaving the individual to make a personal decision on how to interpret them and how to apply them to his own behaviour. Such an approach, concentrating on personal choice, seems a particularly appropriate one from a Christian point of view. Opportunities exist for a statement of personal beliefs and most health educators expect to be asked about their own views.

Some of the subjects in the syllabus are controversial, especially those associated with sexual problems, and the Christian has an important contribution to make. While the prime purpose of teaching sexual development and physiology in schools is to give information about normal functions, the subject cannot be divorced from human relationships and the importance of marriage to a healthy society (see p. 78).

The community physician will usually be involved in discussion of an integrated syllabus with other members of the teaching team. Efforts are made to ensure that the syllabus is as comprehensive as possible and that the ethical problems associated with the subjects are fully discussed beforehand. The use of special visiting lecturers to deal with subjects such as drugs or sexual behaviour without any reference to the health education syllabus as a whole is now generally condemned.

The Family Planning Association – an organization with a long and distinguished history, which has received extensive financial support in recent years from central government – has been particularly active in some areas in providing special teaching in schools concerning contraception and sexual relationships. Not only is the quality of some of this teaching sometimes open to considerable criticism but such sessions are usually based on highly dubious ethical principles. The apparent endorsement of such organizations by the government does not discharge the community physician from his responsibility to ensure that acceptable professional standards in teaching content are maintained and balanced ethical values are conveyed at local level.

The Health Education Council is largely financed by central government to determine wider aspects of health education policy, to organize national campaigns and to produce publicity material for local use. After an unhappy beginning the Council has set a high standard especially in field-testing its literature and posters which are particularly directed at certain sections in the community. Unfortunately, like television commercials, such material has less appeal for professional groups upon whom the Health Service relies for its effective display. While there must be constant vigilance to ensure that the material does not convey unacceptable moral values, doctors should be cautious about rejecting particular posters for what are often essentially aesthetic rather than ethical reasons. Again, the official position of the Council should not be allowed to give any of its material an authority or an approval which it should not possess.

In the wider field of health education, important ethical principles arise. It is generally accepted that there must be some limitation on the freedom of individual choice for the common good, but it is arguable how far the techniques of persuasion employed in advertising and by the media should be used for this purpose. It could be said that there is no threat to individual responsibility in that each person determines the extent to which he is influenced by the message, and the relative ineffectiveness of much advertising, and health education in particular, is apparent to all. The known resistance of consumers to changing brand loyalties suggests an individual assertiveness which might give cause for some satisfaction on the ethical issues involved. However, knowledge in the field of human behaviour is still imperfect, although growing rapidly, and the extent to which individual behaviour can be manipulated is still unknown. While it would seem illogical not to use modern media to transmit the messages of health education, the question must be asked whether it is right to manipulate human behaviour in this way, even though the end may seem justifiable. Such means could just as easily be used to achieve wrong ends.

At present it seems appropriate both from a general ethical and from a Christian viewpoint to support health education and other manipulative programmes directed at large groups of people. The most advanced and sophisticated techniques are acceptable provided that some residual choice is left with the individual. It seems wise, however, to avoid the use of such techniques on a clinical basis and particularly those which effectively deny free choice by offering to an individual only unattractive alternatives.

Relations with Colleagues

The Management of Resources

By definition the work of the community physician should involve him in problems of resource allocation (see p. 154). At a time of economic stringency the discrepancy between wants, needs and resources is magnified and progress in one field can be made only at the expense of another. Many clinicians find it hard to accept the diversion of money from immediate patient care to, say, engineering works in the boiler room or repairs to the roof of the staff canteen, and may accuse the community physician of lacking the ethical standards which are alleged to result from close contact with the realities of patient care. He knows, however, that resources are not unlimited, that some form of rationing is essential[8] and that priorities must be established. For example, he will notice that the majority of patients now treated in the Health Service are elderly, and he may wonder whether some of the surgical and medical treatment they receive is entirely appropriate to their needs or best interests. He cannot avoid the ethical consequences of his decisions, but by defining exactly what the service is trying to achieve, and proposing priorities, he will be able to justify the ethical approach of his decisions and defend them if challenged. Within this framework individual clinical decisions will be made. Clinical freedom must be maintained but it needs to be correctly applied and not used as an excuse to exempt clinicians from the consequences for financial management of the decisions they take.

Equally, the community physician should not acquiesce in the maintenance of conditions which he knows to be professionally intolerable. For example, fire precautions, designed to reduce what has historically been a small risk, are sometimes given priority over measures designed to reduce known and definable medical risks. The fact that the Authority will be responsible for the former risk and the clinician for the latter indicates the dilemma involved and the responsibility that rests on the community physician to support the proper choices.

Increasingly, health services are being seen in economic terms[9] and the new subject of health economics has emerged. It is sometimes suggested that economic considerations demand that priority in health services be given to those who have most to contribute to the community, but this is an unacceptable philosophy. In Western Europe where the Christian influence has been strong, every human being is considered to be equally important, whether young or old, healthy or ill, fit or handicapped. Cost effectiveness is important in assessing the services provided, but should not extend to the point where clinical decisions are infringed. It must also not be confused with cost benefit analyses whose conclusions often depend on a single speculative assumption.

In fact health services are only part of wider considerations of social policy. Policies in areas such as housing, town planning, education and the social services have created many of the problems with which doctors have to deal. If all social policies could be co-ordinated, certain types of ill-health in the community might be prevented. For instance, a progressive taxation system could eliminate smoking as a major health hazard both more effectively and more cheaply than could a health education programme. The concepts of social rewards for healthy behaviour and social punishments for behaviour likely to lead to disease are now being seriously considered. There are not necessarily any ethical implications in these concepts provided that significant areas of free choice and individual responsibility are retained, even though the individual may find himself heavily disadvantaged by choosing certain types of behaviour. The position would be different if the principle were extended to the treatment or non-treatment of certain diseases according to the individual's assumed responsibility for their generation. A doctor is ethically bound to respond to the needs of a patient without consideration of race, nationality, religion or politics. Moral or economic judgements about aetiology do not modify this responsibility.

Review of Services

The community physician is responsible for reviewing the totality of medical services in his area and is likely to find uneven distribution of interest by the medical profession in different medical problems. Services for the acutely ill generally attract greater professional enthusiasm than those for the elderly or the mentally ill, who often have to be cared for in dilapidated buildings with few facilities for investigation and care. Such services also suffer in competition for nursing and other paramedical staff. Yet in numerical terms it is these specialties which present the greatest challenge to the Health Service in the foreseeable future. It is not acceptable for doctors to treat only those patients whose care brings them satisfaction. Rather, the needs of patients should first be ascertained and services adjusted to cater for them. Some hospitals are sometimes reluctant to admit elderly sick or injured folk, since they realize the problems which will arise when these patients are ready for discharge. Care of the aged has always been a particular responsibility readily accepted by the Christian Church and expressed most recently in the field of terminal care. It is disappointing that the most appropriate facilities are often provided outside the Health Service.

Professional Standards

A community physician in the reorganized NHS stands in a unique and privileged relationship with his medical colleagues. He may be charged with the investigation of complaints, with the interpretation of individual terms and conditions of service, and (through the statistics reaching his office) he will be able to assess the quantity, if not the quality, of their work. Additional responsibilities as cremation-referee often provide unexpected insight into local clinical standards. The replies to the statutory questions reveal whether death was anticipated and the degree of medical supervision given in the final illness. Monitoring clinical work is properly the province of clinicians themselves through the medical advisory machinery. In its report *Competence to Practise* the Committee, led by E. A. J. Alment,[10] endorsed this principle unequivocally. There are, however, two ethical points arising in this situation; to what extent is the community physician obliged to take action if the standards he observes are not in accordance with his own, and to what extent is this privileged information, since it arises from the application of medical knowledge to the basic facts put before him?

Area and Regional Medical Officers have a duty to take action upon receipt of a specific complaint under the 'Three Wise Men' procedure (see p. 29).

If a doctor is convicted of an offence in the courts, the community physician should normally report the fact to his Authority. The Department of Health and Social Security has advised Authorities to report such cases to the General Medical Council (GMC) who alone can determine what disciplinary action, if any, is necessary. The Merrison Committee (1975)[11] reported, however, that employing authorities rarely, if ever, notified the GMC of such matters. Some community physicians with responsibilities for personnel may have the duty of suspending or dismissing medical staff on disciplinary grounds.

The community physician would not be wise to ignore unacceptable factors or professional misconduct in the work of a colleague especially if they had an adverse effect on patient care, and at least he should discuss the alleged facts with the colleague concerned and take such action as, in his professional opinion, is required. The Medical Society of New York State (1976)[12] goes further in its principles of professional conduct stating unequivocally that 'A doctor of medicine should expose without fear or favour incompetent, corrupt, dishonest or unethical conduct on the part of members of the profession'.

In all these matters there must be a personal concern for the colleague involved. The full facts of the situation may not be immediately apparent, and the matter should first be discussed in confidence with a senior clinical colleague before further action is taken. The presence of illness in a colleague presents particular difficulties especially if he has no apparent insight into his own condition. Often the community physician will be among the first to be aware of the situation and he should again involve a senior clinical colleague so that the supportive mechanisms advocated by the Alment Committee (1976) can be mobilized quickly.

On the second point, the application of medical knowledge, even to facts that are generally available, is ethically privileged information,

in the same way that many may know that a patient is ill although
none may be aware of the details of the condition or of its treatment.
The circulation of information should be limited to those whose
advice is needed to resolve the matter.

Confidentiality

Traditionally, medical practice has been based on a confidential
relationship between doctor and patient. All information revealed
during a medical consultation has been regarded as confidential and
most doctors find it necessary to record this information. Thus, if
confidentiality is important, it follows that great care must be taken
with the custody of medical records and the information they contain.

Confidentiality may have its origin in the primitive belief that one
who had some intimate knowledge of another possessed a supernatural power over him. There are, however, considerable practical
reasons why confidentiality is still important. Nowadays the medical
relationship is not so unique that it alone creates an ethical reason for
preserving traditional behaviour. Ethical principles can only be
derived from the particular value system adopted in Society. Such
principles are equally applicable to other professional groups whose
members adopt the same values.

In Judaeo-Christian thought there is no specific biblical injunction
on confidentiality but there are a number of principles which give
clear guidance in the matter. It is repeatedly stated that each
person is accountable before God for his acts of omission or commission. In spite of references to the corporate responsibilities of particular communities, the importance of the individual is strongly emphasized. An individual is devalued in his own eyes and in those of his
contemporaries by the publication of intimate details of his life, with
or without his consent. The biographies of famous men are an obvious
illustration of this process. Doctors themselves are often unable to
ensure that their own medical histories remain confidential. When
these become the subject of wider debate the damage to the individual is obvious to all. There are similarities between the medical
relationship and the prayer relationship. In each case there is a
personal dialogue, usually involving only two persons, in which very
personal matters are discussed and action agreed. Christian teaching
emphasizes that prayer is a very private thing and secrecy is posi-
tively encouraged. Finally some illnesses are the result of wrong
actions or imagined wrongs and the doctor and the patient must
jointly face the facts and come to terms with them. If such information reached a wider audience, the patient would continually be
reminded of these circumstances whereas the Bible specifically urges
repentance followed by final and complete forgiveness.

A continuing practice of confidentiality in the doctor-patient relationship can, therefore, be derived from Christian teaching and it

offers practical advantages. The patient can put his full trust and confidence in the doctor if he knows that information passing between them will not be revealed elsewhere. A wide range of matters which many still regard as 'private' must often be explored if the patient's problems are to be identified. Anything which inhibits a patient's willingness to provide this information reduces the help which the doctor can give. Moreover, human relationships on this earth seem to depend on a certain level of secrecy concerning individual thoughts and actions. Indiscriminate dissemination of information can only disturb such relationships and may make the final position of the patient worse than when he first sought help. These principles apply not only to doctors. Other counsellors today enjoy similar privileges, but, unlike doctors, they mostly lack a long established traditional pattern. The need for these professions to codify their ethical practices with appropriate enforcement sanctions is most urgent.

It should be noted, however, that the arguments put forward give no basis for the traditional practice of withholding information from the patient. Indeed they tend to emphasize the need for the patient to be told both the diagnosis and the cause of his condition in terms which he can understand unless there are very powerful reasons to the contrary.

Administrative Work The community physician's work involves the analysis and interpretation of numerical data, much of it relating to individual patients or to doctors and other professional staff within the Service. He is responsible for seeing that the information does not identify individual patients to others, and is not given to other bodies, such as research agencies, without the knowledge and consent of the patient. The Medical Research Council has demonstrated, however, that the need for such consent could be potentially damaging to legitimate research enquiries (Alment 1976) and is developing a code of practice suitable for general application (see p. 175). The security of medical records is likewise the province of the community physician. He must never assume that information in his possession can be freely circulated, even though he may believe it to be common knowledge or information which most patients would not consider to be private. The fact that a person is healthy is confidential medical information since, if the healthy can be identified in a defined population, then illness can be assumed in the remainder.

If information is being handled by non-medical staff the community physician must see that staff receive adequate guidance concerning confidential matters. If ethical standards are to be maintained when the staff changes, a written code of practice will be required to which all are asked to assent at the time of recruitment. Disciplinary action may be necessary in the event of non-compliance and written procedures will certainly be necessary if such action is to be effective.

There is much slackness even among doctors in the abuse of the terms 'private and confidential' or 'personal' on correspondence, and a more uniform practice for each hospital would be a major advance. Even the basic principles of checking the name and credentials of telephone callers before releasing information should be regularly applied. Standards of confidentiality are undoubtedly being eroded because the practical consequences of their systematic application are time-consuming and inconvenient. Whatever system is applied it needs to be regularly checked; although this is accepted for fire precautions, staff often seem to regard a check of confidentiality arrangements as unwarranted interference. Some issues present special problems and are now considered.

Vaccination and Immunization Records   It is customary to record details of date, site of administration and batch number at the time of the procedure, although the only information required after a few weeks is the fact of the immunization and the date on which it was given. Such information is now stored in computer files and many would regard it as no longer confidential although by definition it is. The community physician needs to consider his attitude towards such records and whether less rigorous criteria can be applied to them than to other forms of medical record.

Medical Appointments   Some patients are embarrassed by receipt of an open postcard summoning them to a medical appointment, even though the number of people to whom this information is broadcast must be very small. This erosion of confidentiality could easily be avoided by the use of a sealed window envelope.

Multi-Disciplinary Teams   The nature of teamwork in the medical and social field means that a doctor will reveal some of the secrets of his patient to other members of the team over whom he has no control. The Seebohm Report (1968)[13] was very critical of doctor's attitudes to confidentiality and seemed to imply that they were too restrictive. Discussions have taken place since that time concerning the establishment of ethical codes for all those who are involved in multi-disciplinary teamwork although even this will not resolve the basic medical dilemma. It is a salutary warning that many doctors find increasing difficulty in keeping their own illnesses confidential especially if they elect to be treated by local colleagues.

Management Teams   These bodies may have to decide whether individual patients should be provided with agency services because no local facilities exist. Most teams insist on full information being made available to all members, although they have no clinical responsibility for the patient. This demand can usually be met by restricting the identification of the patient to his initials and part of his address.

Medical Recommendations for Re-Housing Local Authority Councillors may argue that they cannot effectively deal with such applications without a detailed understanding of the medical background. The ethical situation of the community physician is complex. He has no professional relationship with the patient and may feel compelled to recommend a course of action contrary to that suggested by the information with which he has been supplied. The clinician may reveal medical facts to the community physician which he would not divulge to non-medical personnel. The community physician must then decide what is transmitted to another source in the patient's best interests and he is ethically accountable for the decisions he makes. In other circumstances, however, the clinician may complete a form which is obviously intended for wider non-medical circulation as a means of executing an earlier clinical decision. When such a document is forwarded to the community physician his task is to interpret it to the organization to whom it is primarily directed and not to exempt the clinician from his own ethical responsibility for the confidential nature of any information so conveyed.

Child Abuse Following a series of well publicized incidents of child abuse, a study group (Franklin 1973)[14] made several recommendations including a proposal that all such children attending casualty departments should have health visitor follow-up. Area Review Committees were established to consider prevention and treatment (DHSS 1976)[15] and many have now created central registers of families considered to be at risk of injuring their children. Factors likely to be associated with high risks are well documented (Baldwin & Oliver 1975).[16] Area Review Committees have now been instructed to establish such registers with information collected from such diverse sources as casualty departments, general practitioners, police records, social services departments and education departments. The families concerned are unaware of the registers and criteria for admission have hitherto not always been clear.

In support of such a procedure it has been argued that the doctor's responsibility is to the child and not to his parents, and that the requirements of secrecy in respect of information given by the parents are therefore secondary. While the view is understandable, its application challenges the ultimate purpose of medical confidentiality which is to encourage the transmission of all relevant information from patient to doctor. Other consequences of central registers are equally serious. Their existence and criteria for admission should be publicly known and such knowledge may result in a reluctance by parents to present seriously injured children to casualty departments at an early stage. The Report on Child Health Services (1976)[17] extends these ethical considerations by recommending that representatives of the State should have powers to intervene on behalf of the child in a variety of circumstances in which the parents are considered to be withholding consent unreasonably. Such an ethical position is at variance with the Report's declared intention to base future child care firmly within the family, and demonstrates how easily standards can be eroded when principles are not clearly determined.

The creation of integrated registers involving other social agencies so that the latter have free access to them constitutes a major departure from the principle that medical information should remain under medical supervision and control and must therefore be firmly challenged. If confidentiality is to remain an essential ethical principle of medical practice, records should not be transferred beyond medical control without the consent of the patient and the doctor to whom the information was originally entrusted.

Occupational Health Records   Modern occupational health services in industry are firmly based on the principle that health records are confidential. Both the employee and the employer can consult the service in the certain knowledge that information from one will not be disclosed to the other except by specific consent. Only as they are seen to be independent of management can such services hope to gain from all employees the respect upon which their effectiveness depends. Community physicians have responsibility for a number of occupational health services in the public sector especially within the National Health Service, for local authorities and certain aspects of the health of teachers and students. When approaching the responsible clinician, the community physician should always make it clear why the request is being made and the likely destination of any information supplied. If an individual chooses to withhold details of relevant health factors from his University or his employer the community physician has no right to overrule that decision but he does have a duty to emphasize in the clearest possible terms to the individual the full consequences which may result from that action. It is often in the individual's own interest that an employer – or educational institution – should take action under health regulations rather than disciplinary regulations but this choice must ultimately rest with the individual concerned. In practice individuals seem unusually willing to volunteer health information and it is not uncommon for quite intimate details to be sought and supplied at a selection interview when no question of medical involvement has arisen.

Summary

The ethical dilemmas in preventive and community medicine are different in nature from those which confront a clinician and his patient. The community physician seeks to balance the needs of the individual against the needs of society at large. In Christian thinking emphasis upon individual accountability is balanced by corporate responsibility. There is clear instruction to seek after righteousness and to guard against any encroachment by the State which would deny the individual's freedom of conscience. Such an encroachment is always insidious and individuals will vary in their perception of the point at which there must be resistance whatever the cost. In a nationalized health service with increasing state domination there is an ever present danger that doctors and other health care workers may compromise traditionally held ethical values by an uncomprehending acceptance of centrally directed policies or by a wrong assumption that their personal misgivings are not shared by others. There is an urgent need for doctors to re-examine traditional assumptions to determine which no longer have any ethical validity and which have already been dangerously eroded to the point where they no longer constitute a sound ethical system. Such an analysis is no less important in the field of preventive medicine and community medicine.

References

1. Godber, G. (1971) *Preventive Medicine in the 70's Chadwick Trust Lecture*. London, Royal Society of Health.
2. DHSS (1972) Report of the Working Party on Medical Administrators. London, HMSO.
3. Buxton, M. J. & West, R. R. (1975) Cost-benefit analysis of long term haemodialysis for chronic renal failure. *British Medical Journal*, **2**, 376–9.
4. Knox, E. G. (1975) Negligible risks to health. *Community Health*, **6**, 244–251.
5. Cochrane, A. L. (1972) *Effectiveness and Efficiency*. London, Nuffield Provincial Hospital Trust. 'R'.
6. Wadsworth, M. E. J., Butterfield, W. H. J. & Blaney (1971) *Health and Sickness: The Choice of Treatment*. London, Tavistock.
7. DHSS (1977) *The Way Forward*. London, HMSO.
8. Cooper, M. H. (1975) *Rationing Health Care*. London, Croom Helm.
9. Card, W. I. & Mooney, G. H. (1977) What is the monetary value of human life? *British Medical Journal*, **2**, 1627–1629.
10. Report (1976) of the Committee of Enquiry into Competence to Practise. (Chairman, E. A. J. Alment) London, Royal College of Obstetricians and Gynaecologists.
11. Report (1975) of the Committee of Enquiry into the Regulation of the Medical Profession. London, HMSO. Cmnd. 6018.
12. Medical Society of the State of New York (1976) Principles of professional conduct. *New York State Journal of Medicine*, **76**, 133–141.
13. Report (1968) of the Committee on Local Authority and Allied Personal Social Services. London, HMSO., Cmnd. 3703.
14. Franklin, A. W. (1973) *Tunbridge Wells Study Group on Non-accidental Injury to Children*. London, Spastics Society.
15. DHSS (1976) *Non-Accidental Injury to Children*. Reports from Area Review Committees Enclosure to LASSL (76) 2 and CMO (76) 2. London, HMSO.

16. Baldwin, J. A. & Oliver, J. E. (1975) Epidemiology and family characteristics of severely abused children. *British Journal of Preventive and Social Medicine.* **29,** 205–221.
17. Report (1976) of the Committee on Child Health Services. London, HMSO. Vol. 1, p. 448, Cmnd. 6684.

13

The Doctor Himself
Douglas Jackson

Many of us have a mental picture of 'The Doctor' although we could not put into words exactly what we think he is like. Some students enter medicine influenced by their memory of the family doctor of their childhood. Most doctors can recall with admiration a past teacher whose patient history taking, thorough examination, reasoned diagnosis or kindness to the patient have been a life-long inspiration.

A picture which vividly captures our imagination is one by Sir Luke Fildes (1844–1927) in the Tate Gallery, London, entitled *The Doctor*. It is old fashioned in that it was painted before the days of laboratory investigations and antibiotics. The Doctor himself was his treatment – he gave his presence and a measure of hope from experience. In the centre of the picture the light falls on the sick child who lies across a couple of chairs in a humble cottage. An oil lamp on the table shines on the doctor's attentive face and on the pale, sleeping features of the child. In the shadows behind stands the anxious father, while the mother sits at another table her face buried in her folded arms. The seated Doctor is deeply concerned for the child lying in front of him. He is anxious, thoughtful yet unhurried. He is probably bewildered and uncertain of the next step he should take to save his patient. Both his clothes and the expectant attitude of the parents reveal his professional authority. Surely there is something he can do? The bottle of medicine on the table, probably a sedative or an antipyretic, portrays both his will to help and the limited resources available to him. However fanciful this Victorian artist's attempt may be, it does immortalize the doctor-patient relationship. Concentration, compassion, dedication, knowledge and humility are all there, but also a slight detachment, arising not from indifference or arrogance, but because the nature of his calling has taught him to face success or disappointment with equanimity. Even today, the doctor himself matters.

The personality of the doctor does not necessarily spell success in medicine. By nature he may be enthusiastic and encouraging, he may be ponderous, gruff and reassuring, he may be reserved yet sympathetic. We remember the extremes and may laugh at them good humouredly. But character is different and is something we admire and covet. It defines the habits and manner of living to which a doctor has committed himself. It is acquired over the years.

Medicine as Service

The practice of medicine is a service, not an academic study. Although it can be given freely it is usually bounded by some sort of contract, whether financed privately, or by insurance, or by the State. In the Western World doctors have always insisted on an independent doctor-patient relationship, whatever the method used to pay the bill, and this has enabled them to keep first their patients' interests and enjoy their trust. Service is not servile; it is not servitude. Some may conceive of the position of the doctor as being debased if his practice is regarded as service. In no way is this true. There is no conflict here with being leader, friend and adviser.

Such was the doctor's profession in the past. He professed to give an expert service to the sick, whatever may have been his motive for starting medicine in the first place. For many doctors and nurses, sharing a common humanity with the sick was a sufficient incentive to tend and to mend. In Western Europe the Christian tradition provided two extra reasons for accepting the serving role – the command of Christ to follow Him in serving rather than being served and His example in healing the blind, the deaf, the paralytic, the epileptic, the mentally deranged, and the lepers during His public ministry.

Science and Compassion

If medical practice is a service, compassion is the dynamic motivation the doctor needs to face the task; his scientific knowledge and skills are his tools for the job. This is true of all aspects of life where we meet one another. For instance, if on a winter's night an elderly driver has a breakdown on a motorway, his desperate hope is that someone with knowledge of cars will be kind enough to stop and help him. Science is the means, compassion is the motive and both together are needed.

There are, of course, secondary motives for medical practice. We have to earn a living and provide for our family, or we may use medical practice for clinical research, or branch off into the corridors of power to be administrators. But we have to beware that the secondary does not become the primary so that the care of the patient suffers.

Those who have the job of selecting students for medical training are often in difficulties in finding out why they want to join the profession and whether they have the right qualities. An applicant for a student place at a certain medical school was asked why he wanted to do medicine. He gave the altruistic answer, 'To help and heal people who are sick'. Apparently this was not appreciated. Candidates were expected to say they wanted to extend scientific knowledge and apply themselves to clinical science. Yet is not this an example of a one-eyed approach to their duties by the selectors? What medicine needs is men and women who are bright enough to master the science, and sensitive enough to want to understand and care for people.

It is true that science and compassion may be uneasy partners in the doctor's life. They are like a pair of spirited horses, and each needs to be kept on a firm rein if they are to pull together in the same harness. The doctor needs both; and each can be looked on as a 'god' by its own particular worshippers. Science is continually changing so the modern doctor needs to be well informed and up-to-date in his reading; but some 'facts' today are discarded hypotheses tomorrow, so for his patients' sake he has to be careful not to be over confident about the latest treatment. The investigator in him must give way to the clinician when the two conflict, and he has to learn that not everything should be done that science has enabled him to do.

In spite of the immense strides made by scientific medicine there are still many conditions for which no cures exist – the lame-brain following head injury, deep facial burns, severe epilepsy, and traumatic paraplegia. Where would we be but for the compassion and sense of duty that compels our medical and nursing colleagues to refuse to abandon these difficult and hopeless cases which they cannot cure. Some of these patients need years of support and personal encouragement. On the other hand, compassion which moves the doctor to help does not make clear what treatment should be given, so it is usually no clear guide to conduct. This is the weakness of our so-called 'compassionate society' which tries to be kind while throwing away the old recognized standards of what is right and true. We need to know clearly what is for a person's good, or we may – with great compassion – do them a serious injury. Too readily we may choose for people the easy way out of their problems and try to remove the inevitable stresses of responsible living. This is not compassion but thoughtless sentimentality.

Respect and Truthfulness

The foundation of medical practice is the consultation – the meeting between the sick, injured or anxious man and the doctor. Two qualities need to characterize this occasion – mutual respect and truthfulness. On the patient's part, there is usually a natural respect for the doctor, especially if he has a free choice of whom he may consult. If, as sometimes happens, he is off-hand or unwilling to talk freely and 'dislikes all doctors', it is probably due to some unhappy previous experience which needs to be brought to the surface and discussed. It may perhaps be part of the clinical picture signifying frustration, vindictiveness or guilt. As doctors we have to learn to listen with the 'third ear' for what the patient is trying to say but perhaps cannot bring himself to mention explicitly – the alcoholic wife, the sex problem, the non-accidental injury. These things are sometimes our business to discover and evaluate. In illness we see people both at their bravest and at their weakest so we are used to making allowance for the exaggeration or the cover-up. But I have never met a patient who expected his doctor to be anything other than straightforward, honest and truthful. The patient and the public expect certain attributes from the doctor, and they will be upset, or go elsewhere, if they do not find them.

The Source of Respect

All our lives, as doctors, we work with people – old and young, rich and poor, bright and subnormal, friendly and aggressive. And yet, when we are busy or preoccupied, it is only too easy to stop thinking of patients as people and to think of them instead as cases, diagnoses, clinical problems or disordered mechanisms. As Paul Tournier has emphasized, 'Our patients want us to know all about their diseases, but they also want to be understood as persons'. Thomas Sydenham, who gave the first classic description of rheumatic chorea in his Medical Observations concerning the History and Cure of Acute Diseases (1668), advised those entering the profession to consider that 'it is no mean or ignoble animal that he deals with. We may ascertain the worth of the human race, since for it's sake God's only begotten Son became man. . . .' Such truths come as a powerful advocacy for humanity in whatever dress we may happen to meet men and women in consultation.

Speaking the Truth

Honesty, truthfulness and the assurance of confidentiality are the basis of the trust which gets patient and doctor off on the same foot together. Of course there is a place for wit and humour, for romancing and small talk, but the serious atmosphere is also needed when the truth is told and the patient knows he is getting it. A patient comes to the doctor to learn the truth about himself not to be fobbed off with half-spoken evasions or obscurities. Often the truth is unpalatable and difficult to tell but it may be harder still to accept. It may be mildly annoying or frankly alarming so that it plunges the patient into acute anxiety or depression. We have to decide how much to tell at one time and how to say it gently. Does the patient want the truth at all? Perhaps not. If we burden him with unpleasant truth we must try to support him and help him to cope with the inevitable reaction. This support usually falls to the general practitioner, the district nurse or the wife (who may sometimes be the best one to break the bad news). There is no rule-of-thumb approach in this difficult aspect of our work because every person is so different. If we withhold the truth it should never be because we fear for ourselves.

Colleagues

No doctor lives to himself; he has his profession to think about. Single-handed practices are becoming fewer every year and doctors in hospital have multiplied. With their colleagues from many other disciplines teamwork is the pattern of modern medical practice. Yet the profession itself is still important and it cannot sink its identity in a general army of healing, caring people. If it does so, rational thought, clear decision-making and the application of medical principles will soon suffer. This is not a defence of elitism. It is rather a restatement of the age long truth that in human affairs leadership is essential. Over the centuries, medical practice has built up a body of knowledge and expertise with an understanding of how it may be effectively applied.

This necessarily has implications for the doctor himself. He needs to keep informed of what his colleagues are doing and thinking in other fields of medicine, particularly where there is advance. He needs too, to be prepared to take the lead, and at times advocate the unpopular course of action – because he knows it is right. Friendly relationships with those around him make communications and action so much easier and more natural. Supporting his colleagues in friendship, in criticism, in discussion, and particularly when they or their families happen to be in personal need, is the hall-mark of a healthy society. And medicine is a small society committed to work for people.

Personal Standards

It is easy when discussing a subject like this to do what Kipling said, to 'look too good or talk too wise', and yet it would be cowardly to omit the subject because of fear of personal failure or of being thought a hypocrite. The doctor's own standards require a life-time study and discipline.

From early times the leaders of the profession have felt the need of a code of morals, such as the Hippocratic Oath or the Geneva Declaration. Such statements are two-edged. Within the profession they are a teaching aid to inform the doctor's conscience about his duties and to strengthen his moral purpose by membership of a group that has this common aim. Outside the profession the codes are an encouragement to the public to have confidence in doctors they have never met before, because they know that these medical standards are widely observed. Medical ethical codes are receiving more attention today than for many years.

Personal standards, however, tend to fall in periods of low morale, and this decade has its special problems in this respect. We doctors have none of us been immune from the general decline. The reason for the low morale is not because doctors, like several other groups, are people under pressure – though this is true. It is not, as some suggest, that they do not like change – change is often stimulating and advances exciting. The reason is that doctors have lost their initiative in the Health Service and those who have taken it over, trained in management, are untrained in medicine or the type of leadership required. As a result hospital organization concentrates on committees, directives, and memoranda instead of on the healing relationships in clinics and at the bedside. The doctor's dedication to do unpaid work at night and at the weekend, because it needs to be done, is still being exploited. Many hospital facilities for work have deteriorated. Those who have worked hard throughout their professional lives to make their own hospitals centres of excellence are told that research and teaching have no place in a new economy where the best should be sacrificed to make standards uniform. Authorities also make decisions, are often unwilling to accept advice from doctors who work with the patients and are disinterested in whether the doctors accept their conclusions. Even in desperate situations, morale can be high when leadership is good; without strong leadership and good communication, human relationships and standards can only deteriorate.

Fortunately, human nature is resilient, and whenever society is walled in by restrictions – by Government, Unions or any other power – some individuals will take wings and fly out over the top. If this breakout is legal, harmless and successful people will be pleased and exhilarated. Sometimes, unfortunately, individuals feel driven by desperation to gain their ends by hurting other people (as in strikes), or by breaking the civil or moral law.

Double Standards

One thing we need especially to guard against and that is the present trend to separate public and private morals. A man may have high professional standards but adopts the attitude that it is unimportant what he does out of hours. 'Professional life is one thing,' he will say, 'but what I do with my free time and private money is my business, and no one else's!' This double standard might be excusable if morality was merely a matter of convenient customs, but it is not. Society can only be held together and effective public service given if there is general agreement about what is right and wrong in human conduct. In addition, moral decisions need to be consistent in whatever setting they are taken. This is what most people mean by integrity – having a clear understanding of what is right and pursuing it without self-interest. If a man is dishonest in his private affairs, can he be trusted with other people's business? A politician may say it does not matter if he lives a promiscuous life or indulges on the side in illicit trading. A business man may think it does not matter if he is an excessive drinker when the day's work is over. But it does. Attitudes and habits shape character, and character influences decision-making whether in public or private. A Home Secretary is unlikely to maintain public standards if his own night-life is flagrantly bad. A headmaster who is unjust and untruthful will not produce honest and fair-minded boys. A doctor who is obsessed with money is not likely to give the extra needed time to patients in the Health Service. The patient *expects* integrity in his doctor and has a right to find it.

Looking to the Future

How should the doctor himself react to the present situation of low morale and financial stringency in the profession?

This is no time for a regretful looking back on a fading world in which things were once better. It is not the time to mourn the loss of Hippocrates disappearing into a shadowy past. It is time to redouble our efforts to produce a higher standard of patient care, even in the more difficult circumstances of the present. If society is sick, are we not supposed to be the physicians? We shall not help by regretting the deterioration we see and silently retreating. Leaders of the past would tell us to be strong and hold fast to the values we believe in, in the confidence that they can be carried through this period of change and uncertainty into the next era of stability. We should look into the future with hope and courage, and continue to advocate the ageless ideals of humanity.

What are ethical values? They include the very things we have discussed in this book. For doctors they include respect for other people without damaging discriminations, not manipulating them to our advantage and always preserving their confidences. They include giving the highest possible standard of care and supporting education and research so that tomorrow's patients will be better treated than today's. These virtues include being efficient and compassionate, truthful and kind, and putting the patient's interests before our own, even when this is to our own disappointment and loss. Merely to know these things is no help; to do them is true wisdom.

Appendix
Codes of Medical Ethics

The statement of code bearing on Medical Ethics which has exerted the widest influence on the university medical faculties and medical colleges of the West is that attributed to Hippocrates, and generally known as the Hippocratic Oath. Several modifications, designed to make it acceptable to the Christian Church and other religions, have been found among mediaeval Mss. The chief modern revision is that adopted at Geneva in 1948 by the General Assembly of the World Medical Association, and known as the Declaration of Geneva.

The follwing is a selection from the more representative of the existing codes and statements, and is intended to supplement the references in the text to the proved need in practice for such guidelines.

  (i) Oath of Hippocrates (6th or 5th Century BC?)
 (ii) Constitution of the World Health Organization (1946)
(iii) Declaration of Geneva and International Code of Medical Ethics of the World Medical Association (1948, revised 1968)
 (iv) Declaration of Helsinki (1964)
  (v) Declaration of Sydney (1968)
 (vi) Declaration of Oslo (1970)
(vii) Declaration of Tokyo (1975)
(viii) Declaration of Hawaii (1977)
 (ix) A Jewish Medical View
  (x) A Christian Medical View
 (xi) Additional Relevant Documents
(xii) Other Religions

(i) The Oath of Hippocrates

I swear by Appollo Physician and Asclepius and Hygieia and Panaceia and all the gods and goddesses, making them my witnesses, that I will fulfil according to my ability and judgement this oath and this covenant:

To hold him who has taught me this art as equal to my parents and to live my life in partnership with him, and if he is in need of money to give him a share of mine, and to regard his offspring as equal to my brothers in male lineage and to teach them this art – if they desire to learn it – without fee and covenant; to give a share of precepts and oral instruction and all the other learning to my sons and to the sons of him who has instructed me and to pupils who have signed the covenant and have taken an oath according to the medical law, but to no one else.

I will apply dietetic measures for the benefit of the sick according to my ability and judgement; I will keep them from harm and injustice.

I will neither give a deadly drug to anybody if asked for it, nor will I make a suggestion to this effect. Similarly, I will not give to a woman an abortive remedy. In purity and holiness I will guard my life and my art.

I will not use the knife, not even on sufferers from stone, but will withdraw in favor of such men as are engaged in this work.

Whatever houses I may visit, I will come for the benefit of the sick, remaining free of all intentional injustice, of all mischief and in particular of sexual relations with both female and male persons, be they free or slaves.

What I may see or hear in the course of the treatment or even outside of the treatment in regard to the life of men, which on no account one must spread abroad, I will keep to myself holding such things shameful to be spoken about.

If I fulfil this oath and do not violate it, may it be granted to me to enjoy life and art, being honoured with fame among all men for all time to come; if I transgress it and swear falsely, may the opposite of all this be my lot.*

(ii) Constitution of the World Health Organization

The States party to this Constitution declare, in conformity, with the Charter of the United Nations, that the following principles are basic to the happiness, harmonious relations and security of all peoples:

Health is a state of complete physical, mental and social well-being and not merely the absence of disease or infirmity.

The enjoyment of the highest attainable standards of health is one of the fundamental rights of every human being without distinction of race, religion, political belief, economic or social condition.

The health of all peoples is fundamental to the attainment of peace and security and is dependent upon the fullest co-operation of individuals and States.

The achievement of any State in the promotion and protection of health is of value to all.

Unequal development in different countries in the promotion of health and control of disease, especially communicable disease, is a common danger.

Healthy development of the child is of basic importance; the ability to live harmoniously in a changing total environment is essential to such development.

The extension to all peoples of the benefits of medical, psychological and related knowledge is essential to the fullest attainment of health.

Informed opinion and active co-operation on the part of the public are of the utmost importance in the improvement of the health of the people.

Governments have a responsibility for the health of their peoples which can be fulfilled only by the provision of adequate health and social measures.

Accepting these principles, and for the purpose of co-operation among themselves and with others to promote and protect the health of all peoples, the Contracting Parties agree to the present Constitution and hereby establish the World Health Organization as a specialized agency within the terms of Article 57 of the Charter of the United Nations.

(iii) International Code of Medical Ethics of the World Medical Association and the Declaration of Geneva

Adopted by the World Medical Association at its General Assembly, Geneva 1948.

* The date of the Hippocratic Oath is not known and views vary between the 6th or 5th Century BC to 1st Century AD. The earliest known Ms., in an unmodified form, is Codex Maxianus Venetus (11th Century), preserved in the Library of St Mark of Venice.

Duties of Doctors in General

A doctor must always maintain the highest standards of professional conduct. A doctor must not allow himself to be influenced merely by motives of profit.

The following practices are deemed unethical: (a) Any self-advertisement except such as is expressly authorized by the national code of medical ethics. (b) Taking part in any plan of medical care in which the doctor does not have complete professional independence. (c) To receive any money in connection with services rendered to a patient other than the acceptance of a proper professional fee, or to pay any money in the same circumstances without the knowledge of the patient.

Under no circumstances is a doctor permitted to do anything that would weaken the physical or mental resistance of a human being except from strictly professional reasons in the interest of his patient. A doctor is advised to use great caution in publishing discoveries. The same applies to methods of treatment whose value is not recognized by the profession. When a doctor is called upon to give evidence or a certificate he should only state that which he can verify.

Duties of Doctors to the Sick

A doctor must always bear in mind the importance of preserving human life from conception. Therapeutic abortion may only be performed if the conscience of the doctor and the national laws permit. A doctor owes to his patient complete loyalty and all the resources of his science. Whenever an examination or treatment is beyond his capacity he should summon another doctor who has the necessary ability.

A doctor owes to his patient absolute secrecy on all which has been confided to him or which he knows because of the confidence entrusted to him. A doctor must give the necessary treatment in emergency, unless he is assured that it can and will be given by others.

Duties of Doctors to Each Other

A doctor ought to behave to his colleagues as he would have them behave to him. A doctor must not entice patients from his colleagues. A doctor must observe the principles of 'The Declaration of Geneva' approved by the World Medical Association.

Declaration of Geneva

(Adopted by W.M.A at its General Assembly 1948, revised 1968).

At the time of being admitted as a member of the Medical Profession: I solemnly pledge myself to consecrate my life to the service of humanity; I will give to my teachers the respect and gratitude which is their due; I will practise my profession with conscience and dignity; The health of my patient will be my first consideration; I will respect the secrets which are confided in me, even after the patient has died; I will maintain by all the means in my power, the honour and the noble traditions of the medical profession; My colleagues will be my brothers; I will not permit considerations of religion, nationality, race, party politics or social standing to intervene between my duty and my patient; I will maintain the utmost respect for human life from the time of conception; even under threat, I will not use my medical knowledge contrary to the laws of humanity. I make these promises solemnly, freely and upon my honour.

(iv) **Declaration of Helsinki**

Recommendations Guiding Doctors in Clinical Research. Adopted by the World Medical Assembly, Helsinki, Finland, 1964

Introduction

It is the mission of the doctor to safeguard the health of the people. His knowledge and conscience are dedicated to the fulfilment of this mission.

The Declaration of Geneva of The World Medical Association binds the doctor with the words: 'The health of my patient will be my first consideration' and the International Code of Medical Ethics which declares that 'Any act or advice which could weaken physical or mental resistance of a human being may be used only in his interest.'

Because it is essential that the results of laboratory experiments be applied to human beings to further scientific knowledge and to help suffering humanity, The World Medical Association has prepared the following recommendations as a guide to each doctor in clinical research. It must be stressed that the standards as drafted are only a guide to physicians all over the world. Doctors are not relieved from criminal, civil and ethical responsibilities under the laws of their own countries.

In the field of clinical research a fundamental distinction must be recognized between clinical research in which the aim is essentially therapeutic for a patient, and clinical research, the essential object of which is purely scientific and without therapeutic value to the person subjected to the research.

I. *Basic Principles*

1. Clinical research must conform to the moral and scientific principles that justify medical research and should be based on laboratory and animal experiments or other scientifically established facts.
2. Clinical research should be conducted only by scientifically qualified persons and under the supervision of a qualified medical man.
3. Clinical research cannot legitimately be carried out unless the importance of the objective is in proportion to the inherent risk to the subject.
4. Every clinical research project should be preceded by careful assessment of inherent risks in comparison to foreseeable benefits to the subject or to others.
5. Special caution should be exercised by the doctor in performing clinical research in which the personality of the subject is liable to be altered by drugs or experimental procedure.

II. *Clinical Research Combined with Professional Care*

1. In the treatment of the sick person, the doctor must be free to use a new therapeutic measure, if in his judgment it offers hope of saving life, reestablishing health, or alleviating suffering.

    If at all possible, consistent with patient psychology, the doctor should obtain the patient's freely given consent after the patient has been given a full explanation. In case of legal incapacity, consent should also be procured from the legal guardian; in case of physical incapacity the permission of the legal guardian replaces that of the patient.
2. The doctor can combine clinical research with professional care, the objective being the acquisition of new medical knowledge, only to the extent that clinical research is justified by its therapeutic value for the patient.

III. *Non-Therapeutic Clinical Research*

1. In the purely scientific application of clinical research carried out on a human being, it is the duty of the doctor to remain the protector of the life and health of that person on whom clinical research is being carried out.
2. The nature, the purpose and the risk of clinical research must be explained to the subject by the doctor.
3a. Clinical research on a human being cannot be undertaken without his free consent after he has been informed; if he is legally incompetent, the consent of the legal guardian should be procured.
3b. The subject of clinical research should be in such a mental, physical and legal state as to be able to exercise fully his power of choice.
3c Consent should, as a rule, be obtained in writing. However, the responsibility for clinical research always remains with the research worker; it never falls on the subject even after consent is obtained.
4a. The investigator must respect the right of each individual to safeguard his personal integrity, especially if the subject is in a dependent relationship to the investigator.
4b. At any time during the course of clinical research the subject or his guardian should be free to withdraw permission for research to be continued.

    The investigator or the investigating team should discontinue the research if in his or their judgment, it may, if continued, be harmful to the individual.

(v) **Declaration of Sydney**

A Statement on Death. Adopted by the World Medical Assembly, Sydney, Australia 1968

The determination of the time of death is in most countries the legal responsibility of the physician and should remain so. Usually he will be able without special assistance to decide that a person is dead, employing the classical criteria known to all physicians.

Two modern practices in medicine, however, have made it necessary to study the question of the time of death further: (1) the ability to maintain by artificial means the circulation of oxygenated blood through tissues of the body which may have been irreversibly injured and (2) the use of cadaver organs such as heart or kidneys for transplantation.

A complication is that death is a gradual process at the cellular level with tissues varying in their ability to withstand deprivation of oxygen. But clinical interest lies not in the state of preservation of isolated cells but in the fate of a person. Here the point of death *of the different cells and organs* is not so important as the certainty that the process has become irreversible by whatever techniques of resuscitation that may be employed. This determination will be based on clinical judgment supplemented *if necessary* by a number of diagnostic aids of which the electroencephalograph is currently the most helpful. However, no single technological criterion is entirely satisfactory in the present state of medicine nor can any one technological procedure be substituted for the overall judgment of the physician. *If transplantation of an organ is involved, the decision that death exists should be made by two or more physicians and the physicians determining the moment of death should in no way be immediately concerned with the performance of the transplantation.*

Determination of the point of death of the person makes it ethically permissible to cease attempts at resuscitation and in countries where the law permits, to remove organs from the cadaver provided that prevailing legal requirements of consent have been fulfilled.

(iv) Declaration of Oslo

Statement on Therapeutic Abortion. Adopted by the World Medical Assembly, Oslo, Norway, 1970

1. The first moral principle imposed upon the doctor is respect for human life as expressed in a clause of the Declaration of Geneva: 'I will maintain the utmost respect for human life from the time of conception.'
2. Circumstances which bring the vital interests of a mother into conflict with the vital interests of her unborn child create a dilemma and raise the question whether or not the pregnancy should be deliberately terminated.
3. Diversity of response to this situation results from the diversity of attitudes towards the life of the unborn child. This is a matter of individual conviction and conscience which must be respected.
4. It is not the role of the medical profession to determine the attitudes and rules of any particular state or community in this matter, but it is our duty to attempt both to ensure the protection of our patients and to safeguard the rights of the doctor within society.
5. Therefore, where the law allows therapeutic abortion to be performed, or legislation to that effect is contemplated, and this is not against the policy of the national medical association, and where the legislature desires or will accept the guidance of the medical profession, the following principles are approved: (a) Abortion should be performed only as a therapeutic measure. (b) A decision to terminate pregnancy should normally be approved in writing by at least two doctors chosen for their professional competence. (c) The procedure should be performed by a doctor competent to do so in premises approved by the appropriate authority.
6. If the doctor considers that his convictions do not allow him to advise or perform an abortion, he may withdraw while ensuring the continuity (medical) care by a qualified colleague.
7. This statement, while it is endorsed by the General Assembly of the World Medical Association, is not to be regarded as binding on any individ-

ual member association unless it is adopted by that member association.

(vii) **Declaration of Tokyo**

Guidelines for medical doctors concerning Torture and Other Cruel, Inhuman or Degrading Treatment or Punishment in relation to Detention and Imprisonment. Adopted by the World Medical Association, Tokyo 1975

Preamble

It is the privilege of the medical doctor to practise medicine in the service of humanity, to preserve and restore bodily and mental health without distinction as to persons, to comfort and to ease the suffering of his or her patients. The utmost respect for human life is to be maintained even under threat, and no use made of any medical knowledge contrary to the laws of humanity.

Declaration

1. The doctor shall not countenance, condone or participate in the practice of torture or other forms of cruel, inhuman or degrading procedures, whatever the offence of which the victim of such procedures is suspected, accused or guilty, and whatever the victim's beliefs or motives, and in all situations including armed conflict and civil strife.
2. For the purpose of this Declaration, torture is defined as the deliberate, systematic or wanton infliction of physical or mental suffering by one or more persons acting alone or on the orders of any authority, to force another person to yield information, to make a confession, or for any other reason.
3. The doctor shall not provide any premises, instruments, substances or knowledge to facilitate the practice of torture or other forms of cruel, inhuman or degrading treatment or to diminish the ability of the victim to resist such treatment.
4. The doctor shall not be present during any procedure during which torture or other forms of cruel, inhuman or degrading treatment are used or threatened.
5. A doctor must have complete clinical independence in deciding upon the care of a person for whom he or she is medically responsible.
6. Where a prisoner refuses nourishment and is considered by the doctor as capable of forming an unimpaired and rational judgment concerning the consequences of such a voluntary refusal of nourishment, he shall not be fed artificially. The decision as to the capacity of the prisoner to form such a judgment should be confirmed by at least one other independent doctor. The consequences of the refusal of nourishment shall be explained by the doctor to the prisoner.
7. The World Medical Association will support, and should encourage the international community, the national medical associations and fellow doctors to support the doctor and his or her family in the face of threats or reprisals resulting from a refusal to condone the use of torture or other forms of cruel, inhuman or degrading treatment.
8. The doctor shall in all circumstances be bound to alleviate the distress of

his fellow men, and no motive – whether personal, collective or political – shall prevail against this higher purpose.

(viii) **The Declaration of Hawaii 1977**

The general Assembly of the World Psychiatric Association has laid down the following ethical guidelines for psychiatrists all over the world.

1. The aim of psychiatry is to promote health and personal autonomy and growth. To the best of his or her ability, consistent with accepted scientific and ethical principles, the psychiatrist shall serve the best interest of the patient and be also concerned for the common good and a just allocation of health resources. To fulfil these aims requires continuous research and continual education of health care personnel, patients and the public.

2. Every patient must be offered the best therapy available and be treated with the solicitude and respect due to the dignity of all human beings and to their autonomy over their own lives and health. The psychiatrist is responsible for treatment given by the staff members and owes them qualified supervision and education. Whenever there is a need, or whenever a reasonable request is forthcoming from the patient, the psychiatrist should seek the help or opinion of a more experienced colleague.

3. A therapeutic relationship between patient and psychiatrist is founded on mutual agreement. It requires trust, confidentiality, openness, cooperation and mutual responsibility. Such a relationship may not be possible to establish with some severely ill patients. In that case, as in the treatment of children, contact should be established with a person close to the patient and acceptable for him or her. If and when a relationship is established for purposes other than therapeutic, such as in forensic psychiatry, its nature must be thoroughly explained to the person concerned.

4. The psychiatrist should inform the patient of the nature of the condition, of the proposed diagnostic and therapeutic procedures, including possible alternatives and of the prognosis. This information must be offered in a considerate way and the patient be given the opportunity to choose between appropriate and available methods.

5. No procedure must be performed or treatment given against or independent of a patient's own will, unless the patient lacks the capacity to express his or her own wishes or, owing to psychiatric illness can not see what is in his or her best interest or, for the same reason, is a severe threat to others. In these cases compulsory treatment may or should be given, provided that it is done in the patient's best interests and over a reasonable period of time, a retroactive informed consent can be presumed, and, whenever possible, consent has been obtained from someone close to the patient.

6. As soon as the above conditions for compulsory treatment no longer apply the patient must be released, unless he or she voluntarily consents to further treatment. Whenever there is compulsory treatment or detention there must be an independent and neutral body of appeal for regular inquiry into these cases. Every patient must be informed of its existence and be permitted to appeal to it, personally or through a representative, without interference by the hospital staff or by anyone else.

7. The psychiatrist must never use the possibilities of the profession for maltreatment of individuals or groups, and should be concerned never to let inappropriate personal desires, feelings or prejudices interfere with the treatment. The psychiatrist must not participate in compulsory psychiatric treatment in the absence of psychiatric illness. If the patient or some third party demands action contrary to scientific or ethical principles the psychiatrist must refuse to co-operate with them. When, for any reason, either the wishes or the best interests of the patient cannot be promoted he or she must be so informed.

8. Whatever the psychiatrist has been told by the patient, or has noted during examination or treatment, must be kept confidential unless the patient releases the psychiatrist from professional secrecy, or else vital common values or the patient's best interest makes disclosure imperative. In these cases, however, the patient must be immediately informed of the breach of secrecy.

9. To increase and propagate psychiatric knowledge and skill requires participation of the patients. Informed consent must, however, be obtained before presenting a patient to a class and, if possible, also when a case history is published, and all reasonable measures be taken to preserve the anonymity and to safeguard the personal reputation of the subject. In clinical research, as in therapy, every subject must be offered the best available treatment. His or her participation must be voluntary, after full information has been given of the aims, procedures, risks and inconveniences of the project, and there must always be reasonable relationship between calculated risks or inconveniences and the benefit of the study. For children and other patients who cannot themselves give informed consent this should be obtained from someone close to them.

10. Every patient or research subject is free to withdraw for any reason at any time from any voluntary treatment and from any teaching or research programme in which he or she participates. This withdrawal, as well as any refusal to enter a programme, must never influence the psychiatrists efforts to help the patient or subject. The psychiatrist should stop all therapeutic, teaching or research programmes that may evolve contrary to the principles of this Declaration.

(ix) A Jewish Medical View

The Hebrew tradition has not adopted a distinctive view of the ethics of medical practice, other than the general implications of the Torah (Law) and the other Sacred Writings. A Declaration, however, was adopted in 1952 for medical students qualifying from the Hebrew University. Historical and detailed information concerning the viewpoints of Judaism in relation to medicine is found in Jakobovits, I. (1975) *Jewish Medical Ethics*. New York, Bloch Publishing Co.

Oath of the Hebrew University (1952)

New Men of Medicine in Israel!
Ye stand this day all of you before your masters in the ways of medicine and its statutes.
That you should enter into covenant with medicine, to fulfill its laws with uprightness, and with all your might and mind.

That there may be established a generation of physicians worthy to do, and faithfully dedicated to succour the sick.

And this covenant which I maketh with you this day saying:—

You are charged night and day to be custodians at the side of the sick man at all times of his need.

You shall watch verily over the life of man even from his mother's womb and let his welfare always be your chief concern.

You will help the sick, base or honourable, stranger or alien or citizen, because he is sick.

And you shall seek to fathom the soul of the sick, to restore his spirit, through understanding and compassion.

Do not hasten to bring forth judgement, and weigh your advice on a wise balance, tried in the crucible of experience.

Be true to him who puts his trust in you. Reveal not his secret and go not about as a talebearer.

And make wise your heart to the well-being of the many, to bring healing for the ailments of the people.

Give honour and esteem to your teachers who have striven to lead you in the paths of medicine.

Increase wisdom, and weaken not, for wisdom is your life and out of it are issues of life.

Be heedful for the honour of your brothers as in honouring them you will yourselves be honoured.

The words of this covenant are most nigh unto you. They are in your mouths and hearts that you may do them and you will all answer – Amen!

Amen, so will we do.

May your efforts to enhance the heritage of medicine in Israel grow and multiply.

(x) A Christian Medical View

The Early Church, and subsequently the Mediaeval Church, modified the Hippocratic Oath, e.g. by substituting the Divine Name for the pagan deities and in other ways appropriate to Christian teaching. In subsequent centuries, prominent physicians, such as Thomas Browne, Thomas Sydenham and Thomas Percival (and many in the nineteenth Century) wrote in advocacy of the application of Christian principles to medical practice. A recent example of the views expressed will be found in an Affirmation by the Christian Medical Fellowship 1975.

Christian Ethics in Medical Practice

Introduction

Medical practice demands more from the doctor than the accumulated knowledge and technical skills handed down from the past. One who is a Christian will wish to be guided, in his personal relations and attitude to work, by the ethical teaching of Christ as recorded in the Bible. Central in this stands His unequivocal and far-reaching summary of the Moral Law – 'Love the Lord your God with all your heart, with all your soul, with all your mind and with all your strength ... and love your neighbour as yourself.' Mark *12*, 30, 31.

Some implications of this principle for the doctor are outlined in the following affirmation. No Christian, however, can hope to meet such a standard except on the basis of his redemption and reconciliation to God in Christ, and by the power of the Holy Spirit in his daily life.

Christ further taught His disciples: 'I am come that they may have life, and have it more fully'. 'It is more blessed to give than to receive.' 'Freely you have received, freely give.' We are accountable to God in all we do and, therefore, we shall endeavour to conduct our private and professional lives in accordance with the standards of Christ:

In Relation to Human Life

1. To acknowledge that God is the Creator, the Sustainer and the Lord of all life.
2. To recognize that man is unique, being made in the 'image of God', and that he cannot be healthy in body and mind unless he lives in harmony with the natural world around him, which he neither ignores nor exploits.
3. To promote a sense of vocation in the work by which men serve one another, and to honour and recommend the Creator's rule of one day's rest in seven.
4. To maintain the deepest respect for individual human life from its beginning to its end, including the unborn, the helpless, the handicapped and those advanced in age.
5. To uphold marriage as a lasting bond, being the divinely appointed means for the care of children, the security of the family and the stability of society.
6. To recognise that sexual intercourse is intended by God only for the marriage relationship and, hence to advocate premarital continence and marital fidelity.

In Relation to Patients

1. To give effective service to those seeking our medical care irrespective of age, race, creed, politics, social status or the circumstances which may have contributed to their illness.
2. To serve each patient according to his need, subordinating personal gain to the interest of the patient and declining to take part in collective action which would harm him.
3. To respect the privacy, opinions and personal feelings of the patient and to safeguard his confidences.
4. To speak truth to the patient, as he is able to accept it, bearing in mind our own fallibility.
5. To do not harm to the patient, using only those drugs and procedures which we believe will be of benefit to him.
6. To maintain as a principle that the doctor's first duty is to his patient whilst fully accepting our duty to promote preventive medicine and public health.

In Relation to Colleagues

1. To deal honestly with our professional and administrative colleagues and

to fulfil those just requirements of the State, which do not conflict with these basic ethical standards.
2. To work constructively with colleagues in scientific research and in training doctors, nurses and paramedical workers, for the benefit of individual patients and the advance of health care throughout the world.

(xi) **Additional Relevant Documents**

Other Declarations and Statements bear upon Medical Ethics. *The Universal Declaration of Human Rights* (obtainable from the United Nations Office of Public Information) was adopted on December 10, 1948 and contains statements which have medical relevance. Following the Nüremberg trials in 1946–49 a statement, subsequently known as the Nüremberg Code, as adopted by the World Medical Association in 1954. It formulated points concerning Experimental Research on Human Beings and is obtainable from the W.M.A.

A number of Medical Institutions and the official bodies for medical research in various countries have issued Reports and Memoranda for the guidance of the writers whose work they support. For example, the (British) Medical Research Council in 1962–63 issued such guidelines in its Report (Cmnd. 2382, pp. 21–25) and this has subsequently been several times amended.

(xii) **Other Religions**

In the late nineteenth and twentieth Centuries many members of the world's great religions have been trained in Western Medicine. In recent times their numbers practising in English-speaking countries has greatly increased. Some of the religions of Asia have medical traditions stretching far into the past. There were certain Codes, appropriate to the prevailing religion such as The Oaths of the Hindu Physician (taken from 'the Susruta') the Chinese Code from 'The Canon of Medicine' (Han dynasty 200 BC – AD 220), 'The Five Commandments of Chen Shih-Kung' (early 17th Century).

Reference to the literature of India, China and Islamic Countries no doubt shows similar developments, influenced by the respective religions, professional, and cultural outlook of the various peoples.

Index

Diseases and disorders are indicated by *italic*.

DATE DUE